Fast Facts

Fast Facts:
Inflammatory
Bowel Disease

Third edition

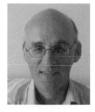

David S Rampton DPhil FRCP
Gastroenterology Clinical Academic Unit
Institute of Cell and Molecular Science
Barts and The London School of Medicine and Dentistry
Queen Mary, University of London
London, UK

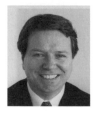

Fergus Shanahan MD
Alimentary Pharmabiotic Centre
Department of Medicine
University College Cork
National University of Ireland
and Cork University Hospital
Cork, Ireland

Declaration of Independence
This book is as balanced and as practical as we can make it.
Ideas for improvement are always welcome: feedback@fastfacts.com

HEALTH PRESS

Fast Facts: Inflammatory Bowel Disease
First published 2000; second edition 2006
Third edition September 2008; reprinted June 2009

Text © 2008 David S Rampton, Fergus Shanahan
© 2008 in this edition Health Press Limited
Health Press Limited, Elizabeth House, Queen Street, Abingdon,
Oxford OX14 3LN, UK
Tel: +44 (0)1235 523233
Fax: +44 (0)1235 523238

Book orders can be placed by telephone or via the website.
For regional distributors or to order via the website, please go to:
www.fastfacts.com
For telephone orders, please call +44 (0)1752 202301 (UK and Europe),
1 800 247 6553 (USA, toll free), +1 419 281 1802 (Americas)
or +61 (0)2 9351 6173 (Asia–Pacific).

Fast Facts is a trademark of Health Press Limited.

The publisher and the authors have made every effort to ensure the accuracy of this
book, but cannot accept responsibility for any errors or omissions.

For all drugs, please consult the product labeling approved in your country for
prescribing information.

A CIP record for this title is available from the British Library.

ISBN 978-1-905832-46-0

Rampton DS (David)
Fast Facts: Inflammatory Bowel Disease/
David S Rampton, Fergus Shanahan

Medical illustrations by Dee McLean, London, UK.
Typesetting and page layout by Zed, Oxford, UK.
Printed by Latimer Trend & Company Limited, Plymouth, UK.

Text printed with vegetable inks on biodegradable and recyclable
paper manufactured using elemental chlorine free (ECF) wood
pulp from well managed forests.

FSC

Mixed Sources
Product group from well-managed
forests and other controlled sources

Cert no. SGS-COC-005493
www.fsc.org
© 1996 Forest Stewardship Council

Glossary of abbreviations

5-ASA: 5-aminosalicylate

ASCA: anti-*Saccharomyces cerevisiae* antibody

ATI: antibodies to infliximab

BMI: body mass index

CARD15: caspase-activiting recruitment domain, member 15 (also known as NOD2)

CDAI: Crohn's Disease Activity Index

CMV: cytomegalovirus

COX: cyclo-oxygenase

CT: computed tomography

CUTE: colitis of uncertain type or etiology

ERCP: endoscopic retrograde cholangiopancreatography

ESR: erythrocyte sedimentation rate

HACA: human antichimeric antibodies, now known as ATI

HLA: human leukocyte antigen

IBD: inflammatory bowel disease

IFN: interferon

IL: interleukin

MAP: mitogen-activated protein

MDP: muramyl dipeptide

MHC: major histocompatibility complex

MP: mercaptopurine

MRI: magnetic resonance imaging

NF: nuclear transcription factor

NF-κB: nuclear [transcription] factor κB

NOD2: other name for *CARD15*

NSAIDs: non-steroidal anti-inflammatory drugs

pANCA: perinuclear antineutrophil cytoplasmic antibody

PPAR: peroxisome proliferator-activated receptor

PPD: purified protein derivatives (prepared from *Mycobacterium tuberculosis* for the Mantoux test, which indicates past or present exposure to tuberculosis)

SeHCAT: ^{75}selenium-labeled homocholic acid taurine

TB: tuberculosis

^{99}Tc-HMPAO: ^{99}technetium-labeled hexamethylpropyleneamine oxime

TGF: transforming growth factor

Th: T helper cell

TNF: tumor necrosis factor

TPMT: thiopurine methyltransferase

Treg: regulatory T cells

Introduction

Inflammatory bowel disease (IBD) comprises two idiopathic chronic relapsing and remitting inflammatory disorders of the gastrointestinal tract: ulcerative colitis and Crohn's disease. Ulcerative colitis affects only the colon and rectum, while Crohn's disease may involve any part of the digestive tract from mouth to anus.

Over recent decades, the incidence of IBD, particularly Crohn's disease, has been steadily increasing; it now affects almost 1 in 250 people in Europe and the USA. Onset is most common in early adulthood, and the chronic waxing and waning nature of ulcerative colitis and Crohn's disease means that together they represent a substantial burden of sickness, not only in hospitals, but also in the community. Because of the wide-ranging effects of IBD, multidisciplinary care of affected patients, both within and outside hospital, is essential.

This third edition of *Fast Facts: Inflammatory Bowel Disease* encompasses recent developments relating to the cause, investigation and management of IBD. We have aimed the book at non-specialist doctors (particularly primary care providers and hospital doctors in training), nurses, stoma therapists, dieticians, psychologists, counselors, social workers and other professionals involved in the care of patients with IBD. Medical students should also find it helpful. We hope too that patients with IBD may benefit from reading this overview of their chronic illness.

The cause of IBD remains unknown, but increasing evidence suggests that these conditions, like many other chronic inflammatory disorders, involve immune-mediated tissue damage due to a variable interaction amongst genetic susceptibility factors and environmental triggers or modifiers (Figure 1.1).

Different mechanisms may account for subsets of disease. For example, various genetic polymorphisms of proteins which sense, or otherwise interact with, the microbial environment in the gut have been shown to predispose to Crohn's disease. This seems to be consistent with the proposal that the disease results, at least in some individuals, from an inappropriate immunologic response to the normal commensal microbiota. However, molecular analysis of the gut microbiota has raised the possibility that a subset of patients with Crohn's disease or ulcerative colitis have an abnormal or altered microbial composition in the gut.

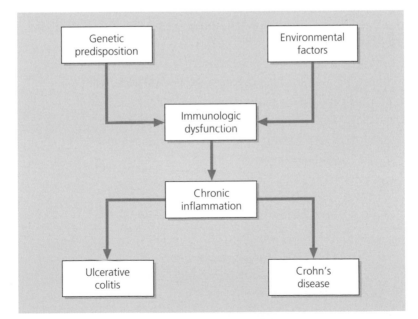

Figure 1.1 Overview of the etiopathogenesis of IBD.

While it remains possible that a specific IBD-causing pathogen is waiting to be discovered, work from several research groups has linked Crohn's disease with a virulent form of enteroadherent *Escherichia coli*. Furthermore, there is intriguing evidence linking defective innate immunity with an altered microbiota. Finally, the complexity of host–microbe interactions in the gut is shown by the finding that some microbial products are protective against pathogenic inflammation whereas others represent an essential ingredient for the pathogenesis of intestinal inflammation in animal models.

Epidemiology

Incidence and prevalence figures for ulcerative colitis and Crohn's disease are shown in Table 1.1. Both diseases are more common in the Western world than in Africa, Asia or South America. However, the incidence of IBD seems to increase in developing countries as they become more westernized. A consistent pattern has been the appearance of ulcerative colitis first, followed by the emergence of Crohn's disease.

Studies of migrant populations from low- to high-prevalence areas confirm the influence of environmental and lifestyle factors, and suggest that their impact is greatest at the earliest stages of life, perhaps while the immune system is still developing. This phenomenon may be due to a variety of factors which may alter the commensal microbiota or influence immune development: these include enhanced sanitation, exposure to antibiotics, vaccination and altered age at exposure to enteric infections. In the West, the incidence of Crohn's disease in particular has risen over the last 40 years, though it may now have leveled off in some countries.

TABLE 1.1

Incidence and prevalence of IBD in the Western world

	Incidence (new cases/100 000 population/year)	Prevalence (cases/100 000 population)
Ulcerative colitis	10	150
Crohn's disease	7	100

Both diseases are slightly more common in women and show a bimodal age distribution, with a major peak at 20–40 years of age and a lesser one at 60–80 years. Jewish and Asian people resident in the USA and UK are more likely to be affected by IBD than those living in Israel and Asia, respectively, confirming that environmental factors are a likely cause. There is no association with social class, but smoking is much more common in patients with Crohn's disease than in those with ulcerative colitis.

Genetic factors. The genetics of IBD is a growth area of research. The identification of the first susceptibility gene for Crohn's disease in 2001, nucleotide-binding oligomerization domain containing 2 (*NOD2*), also known as *CARD15* (caspase-activating recruitment domain family, member 15), prompted an intense search for additional genes. This has been facilitated by several technological advances, particularly the advent of genome-wide association scans. In addition, insights into disease mechanisms arising from different underlying genetic defects have been acquired from a diversity of genetically engineered mouse models, most of which involve defective mucosal barrier function or defective immune regulation. From human and experimental studies, the following generalizations may be made.

- Genetic factors are more important in Crohn's disease than in ulcerative colitis (Table 1.2).
- No single susceptibility gene is either necessary or sufficient to lead to disease.
- Multiple genes are involved, leading to extensive disease heterogeneity.
- Different mechanisms may lead to similar phenotypes.
- Gene–gene interactions modify the severity of disease. For example, susceptibility to inflammatory disease caused by a single genetic defect in mice varies depending on the background strain.
- Gene–environment interactions are confirmed by the requirement for enteric bacteria for full development of disease in animal models.
- Distinct genetic susceptibility factors may underlie Crohn's disease confined to the colon (i.e. factors distinct from those underlying small-bowel Crohn's disease).

TABLE 1.2

Genetic factors in the etiology of inflammatory bowel disease

Factor	Ulcerative colitis	Crohn's disease
Epidemiology		
Prevalence in first-degree relatives	5%	10%
Concordance in monozygotic twins	10%	40%
Ethnic differences in prevalence*	Yes	Yes
Disease associations (e.g. ankylosing spondylitis, Turner's syndrome)	Yes	Yes
Genetic associations		
MHC linkage	Yes	Yes
IBD1, NOD2	No	Yes
ATLG 16L1 and *IRGM*	No	Yes
Chromosome 5q31 (*IBD5*)	No	Yes
IL23R	Yes	Yes
IL12B	Yes	Yes
NKX2-3	Yes	Yes
MST1	Yes	Yes
ECM1	Yes	No
Disease markers		
Increased gut permeability	Yes	Yes
Defective colonic mucus	Yes	–
Altered immune regulation	Yes	Yes
pANCA	Yes	–
ASCA	–	Yes

*More common in Ashkenazi than Sephardic Jews and more common in North American whites than in African Americans.

ASCA, anti-*Saccharomyces cerevisiae* antibody; *ATLG 16L1*, autophagy-related 16-like 1 gene; *ECM1*, locus encoding extracellular matrix protein 1; *IL12B*, gene encoding interleukin-12b; *IL23R*, gene encoding interleukin-23 receptor; *IRGM*, immunity-related GTPase family, M; MHC, major histocompatibility complex (chromosome 6, includes human leukocyte antigen [HLA] loci); *MST1*, macrophage-stimulating 1; *NKX2-3*, NK2 transcription factor related; *NOD2*, nucleotide-binding oligomerization domain containing 2; pANCA, perinuclear antineutrophil cytoplasmic antibody.

- Many of the susceptibility genes identified for Crohn's disease are involved either in the sensing or intracellular processing of bacteria (innate immunity) or in immune regulation.
- Most genome-wide association scans have been conducted in populations of European ancestry, but some loci are not associated with Crohn's disease in Japanese people – suggesting that the genetics of Crohn's disease varies across populations.
- Some but not all genetic (and environmental) risk factors are common to ulcerative colitis and Crohn's disease, whereas others are disease-specific (Table 1.2).

Reduced clearance of intracellular bacteria, resulting from *NOD2* or autophagy gene variants, may predispose to Crohn's disease but not to ulcerative colitis, whereas defects in other genes (e.g. the IL-23 receptor gene) are genetic risk factors for both Crohn's and ulcerative colitis, and a defect in the *ECM1* locus (encoding extracellular matrix protein 1) has been shown to predispose to ulcerative colitis (Table 1.2).

NOD2. Two single-nucleotide polymorphisms of and one frame-shift mutation in the *NOD2* gene at the *IBD1* locus on chromosome 16 are associated with a greater than fortyfold increased risk of Crohn's disease for individuals who are homozygous for all three. About 40% of European patients with familial Crohn's disease carry one of the three *NOD2* mutations. *NOD2* mutations predispose in particular to fibrostenosing small-bowel and right-sided colonic Crohn's disease.

The protein encoded by *NOD2* is an intracellular pattern recognition receptor, a sensor for bacterial peptidoglycan that can be activated by a component of peptidoglycan, muramyl dipeptide (MDP).

The polymorphisms identified may confer susceptibility to Crohn's disease by altering immunorecognition of the constituents of bacterial flora and by modifying activation of the nuclear [transcription] factor NF-κB (nuclear factor κB). However, because *NOD2* mutations account for only 20–30% of cases and are not linked with Crohn's disease in Japanese and others of Oriental descent, this genetic risk factor, like others, is neither necessary nor sufficient for the development of Crohn's disease.

Autophagy-related gene defects. Autophagy (self-eating) is a normal cellular event in the homeostatic control of growth and development by which cellular components are degraded or recycled. It is also central to the processing of intracellular pathogens. Variants in the autophagy-related 16-like 1 gene (*ATLG 16L1*) and the *IRGM* gene (immunity-related GTPase family, M) have been confirmed as genetic susceptibility factors for Crohn's disease but not ulcerative colitis. The resulting increased intracellular bacterial load may lead to the secondary Th1 activity within the mucosa that characterizes Crohn's disease.

Interleukin-23 receptor (IL-23R). Several polymorphisms of the gene encoding IL-23R have been linked with Crohn's disease (conferring protection or risk), and also contribute to the risk of ulcerative colitis. IL-23 is a pivotal cytokine in the generation of Th17 effector cells and interleukin-17 (IL-17), which contribute to chronic mucosal inflammatory disease, particularly Crohn's disease.

The ECM locus (extracellular matrix protein 1) has recently been identified as a susceptibility locus for ulcerative colitis. The extracellular matrix protein 1 encoded here is a glycoprotein expressed in the small and large bowel that interacts with the basement membrane, inhibits matrix metalloproteinase 9, and can activate NF-κB.

Environmental factors. Epidemiological and other evidence has identified a number of environmental factors that may play a role in the etiopathogenesis of IBD (Table 1.3).

Smoking. Only about 10% of patients with ulcerative colitis smoke, compared with 30% of the normal population and 40% of those with Crohn's disease. A history of recent cessation of smoking is common in patients presenting with ulcerative colitis for the first time, and nicotine patches have a modest therapeutic benefit. Conversely, smoking increases the risk of relapse and of surgery in small-bowel Crohn's disease (although not clearly in colonic Crohn's disease), while cessation improves the natural history of the disease. Nicotine and other constituents of tobacco smoke have a variety of effects on the inflammatory response, but it is not known why these are beneficial in patients with ulcerative colitis yet harmful in those with Crohn's disease. It is possible that the effects of smoking are organ- rather

TABLE 1.3

Environmental factors that may exacerbate IBD

Factor	Ulcerative colitis	Crohn's disease
Cigarettes		
Ex-smokers*	Yes	–
Smoking	–	Yes
Dietary factors	Milk (rarely)	Various
Infection	Enteric infections	Under investigation
Drugs		
NSAIDs	Yes	Yes
Antibiotics	Yes	Yes
Oral contraceptives	Yes	Yes
Other factors		
Appendiceal inflammation[†]	Yes	No
Psychological stress	Yes	Yes

*Cessation of smoking linked to onset of ulcerative colitis.
[†]Appendectomy at an early age is protective against ulcerative colitis.
NSAIDs, non-steroidal anti-inflammatory drugs.

than disease-specific: harmful to small, but protective to large, intestinal mucosa.

Diet. In ulcerative colitis, up to 5% of patients improve by avoiding cows' milk, but no other potentially pathogenic dietary factors are known. Patients with active Crohn's disease improve when their ordinary food is replaced by a liquid formula diet, and they may deteriorate thereafter on the introduction of specific foods (see Chapter 6). However, no particular foods that are universally detrimental to patients with Crohn's disease have been identified. A high-fat diet has been linked with recent increases in the frequency of IBD in Japan.

Specific infection. Despite its resemblance to, and occasional onset after, infective diarrhea, there is no evidence that ulcerative colitis is due to a single infective agent. Neither Crohn's disease nor ulcerative colitis appear to be caused by a transmissible pathogenic infection in the traditional sense. However, several groups have identified a virulent form of enteroadherent *E. coli* in patients with Crohn's disease. Whether this is causal or consequential to defective innate immunity is unclear. Several investigators have suggested that an atypical mycobacterial infection may cause Crohn's disease. The organism, *Mycobacterium paratuberculosis*, does appear to be common in the environment and can occur in the food chain, but a causal link with Crohn's disease is unproven. Earlier claims that measles virus and measles vaccination may predispose to Crohn's disease have been discounted.

Enteric microflora. Resident gut microflora are likely to be a major environmental factor in the pathogenesis of IBD. Circumstantial clinical and direct experimental evidence highlights the importance of the fecal stream in driving mucosal inflammation. The presence of gut flora is required for the full expression of enterocolitis in genetic and induced animal models of IBD. Patients with active IBD show loss of immunologic tolerance to intestinal microflora. Lastly, antibiotics and possibly probiotics have a therapeutic role in IBD.

Drugs. Relapse of IBD may be precipitated by non-steroidal anti-inflammatory drugs (NSAIDs), perhaps as a result of inhibition of the synthesis of cytoprotective prostaglandins, and by antibiotics, probably secondary to changes in enteric flora. The oral contraceptive pill has been associated epidemiologically with Crohn's disease in particular: conceivably, the explanation is vascular.

Appendectomy. Previous appendectomy is rare in patients developing ulcerative colitis: it has been suggested that T cells in an inflamed appendix could trigger inflammation (ulcerative colitis) in the more distal large bowel in genetically predisposed individuals.

Stress. Psychological stress due to the unpleasant, chronic and intractable nature of the illness is common in those with IBD, particularly Crohn's disease. It is possible that, for some people, stress may itself trigger relapse, as has been shown in animal models – for example, by activation of leukocytes by enteric nerve endings in the gut wall (Figure 1.2).

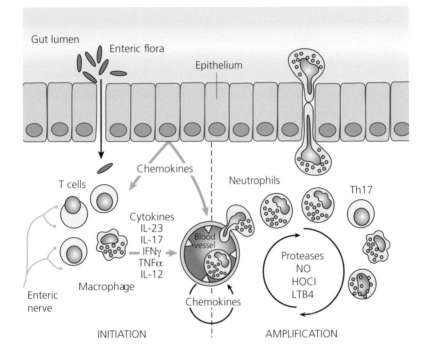

Figure 1.2 Mediators and mechanisms involved in the pathogenesis of IBD. The initiating factors are uncertain, but may include a breakdown in tolerance to enteric flora. T-cell and macrophage activation leads to production of cytokines, which act at several levels, including the local microvasculature. The chemokine gradient generated causes transmigration of neutrophils, leading to tissue damage by metalloproteases and other reactive substances, augmentation of the inflammatory response and disruption of the epithelial barrier, itself causing further ingress of enteric flora and their products. The inflammatory response may be modulated by activation of lymphocytes by enteric nerve endings. HOCl, hypochlorite; IFNγ, interferon γ; IL, interleukin; LTB4, leukotriene B4; NO, nitric oxide; Th17, T helper cell 17; TNFα, tumor necrosis factor α.

Pathogenesis

The initiating factor or factors in IBD are unknown, but there is good understanding of the amplification phase and final common pathway of tissue injury in both forms of the disease.

Upregulation of the expression of nuclear transcription factors, such as NF-κB, underlies the subsequent excessive local release of cytokines, growth factors, reactive oxygen metabolites, nitric oxide, eicosanoids (leukotrienes, thromboxanes and prostaglandins), platelet-activating factor, proteases, neuropeptides and other mediators (see Figure 1.2). Details of these molecular events and the mediators involved are beyond our scope here, but some points of distinction between ulcerative colitis and Crohn's disease are noteworthy.

While there is considerable overlap between the two forms of IBD, the cytokine profile in ulcerative colitis has traditionally and simplistically been described as a non-Th1 pattern, whereas that of Crohn's disease has been considered to be a typical Th1 pattern (Table 1.4). More recently, the Th17 effector cell and associated cytokine profile have been linked with several immune-mediated disorders, including Crohn's disease. This CD4+ T-cell lineage is generated by IL-23, produces IL-17, and is counterregulated in a complex manner by the Th1 and Th2 pathways. The IL-23–Th17 pathway is now under investigation as a therapeutic target in IBD. The balance of effector cells in the mucosa is subject to several regulatory constraints which include regulatory T cells (Treg). In the absence of inflammatory signals, transforming growth factor (TGF)-β tends to promote the development of Tregs which suppress inflammatory responses, whereas in the presence of inflammatory cytokines such as IL-6, TGF-β induces the differentiation of Th17 cells.

The immunologic disturbances in ulcerative colitis include prominent autoimmune responsiveness, whereas those in Crohn's disease appear to be primarily directed against components of the gut microbiota. In both disorders, this might suggest an underlying defect in immune regulation, but evidence for a primary immunoregulatory defect in humans with either disorder remains to be shown.

In contrast, there is compelling evidence for a deficiency in innate immunity, particularly in some patients with Crohn's disease. An increased bacterial load in the mucosa of patients with Crohn's disease has been well demonstrated, and this may be secondary to defective processing of intracellular bacteria (as discussed previously), related to variant genes such as *NOD2* or autophagy genes. Furthermore,

TABLE 1.4

Immune and inflammatory response in inflammatory bowel disease

	Ulcerative colitis	Crohn's disease
Humoral immunity		
Association with autoimmune disease (e.g. Hashimoto's thyroiditis, SLE)	Strong	Weak
Autoantibody production (e.g. anticolon antibody, pANCA)	Common	Rare
Cell-mediated immunity		
Mucosal infiltrate	Non-granulomatous Neutrophils prominent	Granulomatous T cells prominent
T-cell reactivity	Normal/decreased	Increased
Cytokine profile		
Th response	Non-Th1 (IL-10 IL-5, IL-13)	Th17 (IL-23, IL-17, IL-2, IFN, IL-12, TNFα)
Other cytokines	IL-1, IL-6, IL-8	IL-1, IL-6
Innate immunity		
		Altered processing of intracellular bacteria
		Reduced defensins

IFN, interferon; IL, interleukin; pANCA; perinuclear antineutrophil cytoplasmic antibody; SLE, systemic lupus erythematosus; Th, T helper cell; TNFα, tumor necrosis factor α.

deficiency of the transcription factor T-bet in the innate immune system of mice has been shown to lead to an alteration in the microbiota which predisposes them to colitis and can transfer the disease to susceptible hosts. Reduced production of defensins, a group of antimicrobial peptides secreted into the lumen by Paneth cells in the small-bowel epithelium, has also been linked with Crohn's disease and may be a contributory factor. In addition, defective phagocyte function, unrelated to *NOD2* function, has been described in patients with Crohn's disease, lending further support for the concept of an immune deficiency state rather than an immunoregulatory disorder.

Defective colonic mucus (in ulcerative colitis) and abnormal intestinal epithelial permeability (in both forms of IBD) may increase the access of luminal dietary and bacterial products to the mucosa. Impaired availability and metabolism of bacterially derived luminal short-chain fatty acids may adversely affect colonic epithelial function in ulcerative colitis, while in Crohn's disease, a procoagulant diathesis and multifocal granulomatous intestinal microinfarction may occur early in the disease process.

Pathology

The macroscopic and microscopic appearances of the bowel play a key role in the diagnosis of ulcerative colitis and Crohn's disease. Despite their names, ulceration is an early event in Crohn's disease even when mild; it is a late event and related to severe disease activity in ulcerative colitis.

Ulcerative colitis usually begins in the rectum, and either remains there or spreads proximally (Figure 1.3). In severe total ulcerative colitis, the distal ileum ('backwash ileitis') is occasionally involved, but this is not clinically important. In the colon, there is diffuse mucosal inflammation with hyperemia, granularity, surface pus and blood, leading, in severe cases, to extensive ulceration. This heals by granulation to form multiple pseudopolyps.

Microscopically, acute and chronic inflammatory cells infiltrate the lamina propria and crypts (producing crypt abscesses). Crypt architecture is distorted and goblet cells lose their mucin (goblet-cell depletion) (Table 1.5, Figure 1.3). The mucosa is edematous with epithelial ulceration. Biopsies in long-standing total colitis may show dysplasia, in which epithelial cell nuclei are enlarged and crowded, and lose their polarity: carcinoma may supervene.

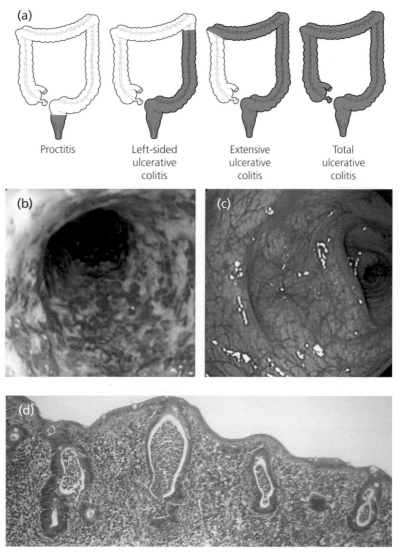

Figure 1.3 (a) Distribution of ulcerative colitis; (b) colonoscopic appearance of active ulcerative colitis – mucopurulent exudate, erythema, granularity and superficial ulceration; (c) normal colonic mucosa for comparison; (d) microscopic appearance of ulcerative colitis – intense inflammatory cell infiltration of the lamina propria, goblet-cell depletion and crypt abscesses. Photomicrograph reproduced courtesy of Professor RM Feakins, Barts and The London School of Medicine and Dentistry, London, UK.

TABLE 1.5

Histology of inflammatory bowel disease

Feature	Ulcerative colitis	Crohn's disease
Lamina propria cell infiltrate	Diffuse, superficial Neutrophils prominent	Discontinuous Deep lymphocytes
Cryptitis, crypt abscesses	Prominent	Focal
Crypt distortion and loss	Widespread	Patchy
Goblet cell mucin depletion	Marked	Rare
Ulceration	Superficial In severe disease only	Superficial (aphthoid) in early disease; deep in later disease
Epithelioid granulomas	None	Occasional

Crohn's disease can affect any part of the gut (Table 1.6). Typically, there are discontinuously affected gut segments (skip lesions). The first visible abnormality is lymphoid follicular enlargement with a surrounding ring of erythema (the 'red-ring' sign); this leads to aphthoid ulceration which, in turn, progresses to deep fissuring ulcers with cobblestoning, fibrosis, stricturing and fistulation (Figure 1.4). Inflammation and fibrosis predispose to intestinal strictures, presenting with obstructing symptoms, and to local perforation of the gut wall, leading to abscess formation.

Histologically, there is transmural chronic inflammatory cell infiltration with ulceration and formation of microabscesses. Non-caseating epithelioid granulomas, sometimes containing multinucleate giant cells, are found in about 25% of patients investigated with colonoscopic biopsies, and in 60% of those examined after surgical resection of the bowel (Table 1.5, Figure 1.5). There is an increased risk of cancer in chronically inflamed areas of small intestinal, anorectal and, particularly, colorectal mucosa.

TABLE 1.6

Sites of Crohn's disease

Site	Proportion of cases (%)
Ileocecal	45
Colitis only	25
Terminal ileum only	20
Extensive small bowel	5
Other (anorectal, gastroduodenal, oral only)	5

Key points – etiopathogenesis

- The most consistent epidemiological clue to etiopathogenesis is the increased prevalence of IBD (ulcerative colitis appearing first, with the later emergence of Crohn's disease) as societies make the transition from developing to developed status. Studies of migrant populations suggest that the risk of IBD may be related to lifestyle or environmental exposure during early life.
- Some genetic and environmental risk factors are common to ulcerative colitis and Crohn's disease and others are disease-specific. Clarification of the genetics of IBD is increasing our understanding of the etiopathogenesis of the disease and highlights defective host–microbe interactions. Genetic investigation promises also to provide crucial information about phenotypic expression of the disease and the likely response to therapy.
- Smoking exacerbates small-bowel Crohn's disease, but it may have a protective effect in ulcerative colitis.
- The histology of affected gut mucosa provides essential clues to the diagnosis of IBD.

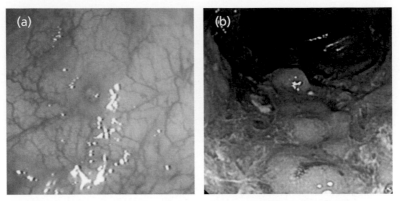

Figure 1.4 Colonoscopic appearances of Crohn's disease: (a) aphthous erosion in early disease; (b) ulceration and 'cobblestoning' in well-established chronic disease.

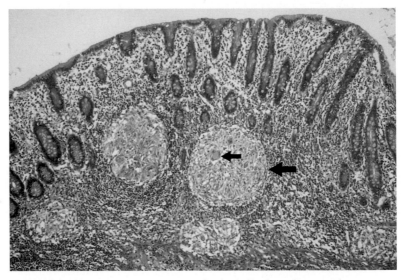

Figure 1.5 Microscopic appearance of colonic Crohn's disease. Three large epithelioid granulomas with multinucleate giant cells are visible; the large arrow shows a granuloma and the small arrow shows a giant cell. Photomicrograph reproduced courtesy of Professor RM Feakins, Barts and The London School of Medicine and Dentistry, London, UK.

Colitis of uncertain type or etiology. In some patients with chronic colitis, the pathological features are not typical of either ulcerative colitis or Crohn's disease. In these people, the term 'colitis of uncertain type or etiology' (CUTE) is preferable to the previously favored 'indeterminate' colitis. 'IBD unclassified' is an alternative term that may be useful in this setting, particularly for those in whom the small bowel has not yet been imaged.

Key references

Cho JH. The genetics and immunopathogenesis of inflammatory bowel disease. *Nat Rev Immunol* 2008;8:458–66.

Fisher SA, Tremelling M, Anderson CA et al. Genetic determinants of ulcerative colitis include the *ECM1* locus and five loci implicated in Crohn's disease. *Nat Genet* 2008;40:710–12.

Frank DN, St Amand AL, Feldman RA et al. Molecular-phylogenetic characterization of microbial community imbalances in human inflammatory bowel diseases. *Proc Natl Acad Sci USA* 2007;104: 13780–5.

Garrett WS, Lord GM, Punit S et al. Communicable ulcerative colitis induced by T-bet deficiency in the innate immune system. *Cell* 2007; 131:33–45.

Marks DJ, Harbord MW, MacAllister R et al. Defective acute inflammation in Crohn's disease: a clinical investigation. *Lancet* 2006;367:668–78. Erratum in: *Lancet* 2007;370:318.

Marks DJB, Segal AW. Innate immunity in inflammatory bowel disease: a disease hypothesis. *J Pathol* 2008;214:260–6.

Mathew CG. New links to the pathogenesis of Crohn disease provided by genome-wide association scans. *Nat Rev Genet* 2008;9:9–14.

Mazmanian SK, Round JL, Kasper DL. A microbial symbiosis factor prevents intestinal inflammatory disease. *Nature* 2008;453:620–5.

Rhodes JM. The role of *Escherichia coli* in inflammatory bowel disease. *Gut* 2007;56:610–12.

Sartor RB. Microbial influences in inflammatory bowel diseases. *Gastroenterology* 2008;134:577–94.

Steinman L. A brief history of T(H)17, the first major revision in the T(H)1/T(H)2 hypothesis of T cell-mediated tissue damage. *Nat Med* 2007;13:139–45. Erratum in: *Nat Med* 2007;13:385.

Strober W, Fuss I, Mannon P. The fundamental basis of inflammatory bowel disease. *J Clin Invest* 2007; 117:514–21.

Clinical features of ulcerative colitis

The onset of ulcerative colitis is usually gradual, and its natural history chronic, with relapses and remissions over many years. Between attacks, patients are usually free of symptoms.

The features of active disease depend on the extent as well as the activity of disease. For formal epidemiological and clinical trial purposes, various classifications of ulcerative colitis have been proposed, most recently at a meeting in Montreal in 2005. For routine clinical use, the main features of the disease are as described below.

Acute severe ulcerative colitis most commonly occurs in patients with subtotal or total disease and causes profuse, frequent diarrhea (six or more loose stools per day) with blood and mucus, peridefecatory abdominal pain, fever, malaise, anorexia and weight loss. On external examination the patient is thin, anemic, fluid-depleted, febrile and tachycardic. In those developing toxic megacolon and/or perforation, further deterioration is usually obvious, with sudden worsening of abdominal pain, distension, fever, tachycardia, sepsis and shock.

Moderate active ulcerative colitis is commonly left-sided, causes rectal bleeding and discharge of mucus accompanied by diarrhea (fewer than six loose stools daily), urgency and sometimes abdominal pain. There may be malaise, but examination is usually normal.

Active proctitis causes rectal bleeding and mucous discharge, often with tenesmus and pruritus ani. There may be diarrhea, but the stool is often well-formed. Indeed, many patients with refractory proctitis are constipated (see Chapter 5 for a fuller discussion of refractory proctitis). General health is usually maintained.

Clinical features of Crohn's disease

The symptoms and signs of Crohn's disease depend on the affected site and the predominant pathological process in each patient. As for ulcerative colitis, the Montreal 2005 consensus proposed a classification based on disease site and behavior, but this is rarely used for routine clinical purposes.

Active ileocecal and terminal ileal Crohn's disease patients usually present with pain and/or a tender mass in the right iliac fossa, with or without diarrhea and weight loss. Possible mechanisms of diarrhea include mucosal inflammation, bile-salt malabsorption (see page 131) and bacterial overgrowth proximal to a stricture (Table 2.1). In patients with symptoms predominantly due to inflammation or abscess, the pain tends to be constant, often with fever. In those with small-bowel obstruction, whether due to active inflammation or to fibrosis and stricture formation in the healing phase, the pain is more generalized, intermittent and colicky, and associated with loud borborygmi,

TABLE 2.1

Mechanisms of diarrhea in Crohn's disease

Mechanism	Treatment
Inflammation	Anti-inflammatory drugs
Small-bowel bacterial overgrowth	Antibiotics
Bile-salt diarrhea	Colestyramine
Bile-salt deficiency	Low-fat diet
Lactase deficiency	Avoid lactose
Short-bowel syndrome	See Table 2.2
Internal fistula	Surgery
Antibiotic-related	Stop antibiotics
Intercurrent infection (e.g. *Clostridium difficile*)	Appropriate antibiotic
Other (e.g. irritable bowel syndrome, celiac disease)	As appropriate

abdominal distension, vomiting and eventually absolute constipation. Enterocutaneous fistulas are clinically obvious, but direct questions about pneumaturia and feculent vaginal discharge may be necessary to identify enterovesical or enterovaginal fistulas. Presentation as an acute abdomen, with peritonitis due to free perforation, is rare.

Active Crohn's colitis causes symptoms similar to those of active ulcerative colitis, although frank bleeding is less common. Extraintestinal manifestations are more common in Crohn's disease of the large bowel than of the small bowel.

Extensive small-bowel Crohn's disease. As well as the above symptoms, patients with extensive small-bowel disease may have features of malabsorption, with steatorrhea, anemia and weight loss.

Perianal Crohn's disease is due to fissure, fistula (Figure 2.1) or abscess, and is suggested by perianal pain and/or discharge. It can be quickly confirmed in most by perineal inspection. Although perianal Crohn's disease is often much less uncomfortable than it looks, sigmoidoscopy (see Chapter 3) may be too painful to undertake without sedation or even anesthesia in some patients.

Gastroduodenal and oral Crohn's disease are both very rare. The former presents with upper abdominal pain or dyspepsia, often with anorexia, nausea, vomiting and weight loss, while the latter causes chronic oral ulceration and/or induration.

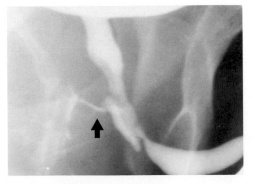

Figure 2.1 Micturating cystogram showing rectourethral fistula in Crohn's disease. The arrow indicates the fistula between the urethra and the rectum.

Intestinal complications of IBD

The main intestinal complications of IBD are undernutrition, short-bowel syndrome and cancer.

Undernutrition. Nutritional deficiency is particularly common in Crohn's disease. Causes include reduced food intake, malabsorption in those with small-bowel disease, increased loss of protein from an inflamed bowel, and increased metabolic requirements in sick patients, including the catabolic effects of cytokines and other inflammatory mediators. Those at particular risk should be monitored carefully for evidence of undernutrition by measurement of weight, at least, and blood tests such as blood count, albumin, folate, vitamin B_{12} (cobalamin), ferritin, calcium and magnesium. Management options range from supplemental sip feeding with appropriate replacement of specific deficiencies, through enteral to parenteral nutrition (see Chapters 5 and 6).

Short-bowel syndrome develops when extensive bowel resection leads to excessive malabsorption of fluids, electrolytes and nutrients. The most common cause is Crohn's disease, but it can also occur with mesenteric vascular occlusion, trauma and neoplasia.

Pathogenesis. Factors influencing symptoms include the extent of resection(s), the presence of residual Crohn's disease and the absence of the ileocecal valve, which normally slows small-bowel transit and inhibits colonization of the distal small bowel by colonic flora. Furthermore, the site of resection is important: terminal ileal resection causes bile-salt malabsorption, vitamin B_{12} deficiency, gallstones and hyperoxaluria, while removal of the colon and small bowel causes severe diarrhea owing to loss of colonic absorptive capacity.

Presentation. Patients present with watery diarrhea immediately after resection. This tends to improve as the intestine adapts, or it may progress to steatorrhea as bile-salt deficiency develops. Later complications include urinary stones and gallstones.

Investigation. Fluid, electrolyte and nutritional deficiencies, stool output, bile-salt malabsorption, vitamin B_{12} absorption and urinary oxalate excretion should be quantified.

Bile-salt malabsorption can be measured by means of SeHCAT scanning; SeHCAT (the taurine conjugate of 23-[75Se]-25-homocholic acid) is a synthetic bile salt that emits gamma rays. After an oral dose, it is absorbed in the terminal ileum, and the amount retained after 7 days can be estimated by whole-body scanning. In patients with extensive ileal disease causing bile-salt malabsorption, retention is usually less than 15%.

Vitamin B_{12} absorption can be measured by the Schilling test. Non-radioactive vitamin B_{12} is injected to saturate the body's stores; 2–6 hours later, radioactive vitamin B_{12} is ingested, with or without intrinsic factor. Urine is then collected over 24 hours to measure the absorption of vitamin B_{12}: reduced urinary excretion after oral administration of vitamin B_{12} with intrinsic factor indicates terminal ileal malabsorption of the vitamin.

Management. Intravenous restoration of fluid and electrolytes and total parenteral nutrition may be necessary at first. Enteral feeding is started early, to promote gut adaptation, using lactose-free iso-osmolar solutions (Table 2.2). Small frequent meals are introduced later, a low-fat diet being helpful for those with marked steatorrhea. Excessive dietary oxalate should be avoided. Loperamide and codeine phosphate may reduce stool output by slowing transit and increasing mucosal absorption.

For patients with extensive small-bowel resections, further treatment options include:

- dietary calorie supplements with medium-chain triglycerides (which are directly absorbed without having to be digested)
- H_2-receptor antagonists or proton-pump inhibitors (to reduce the gastric hypersecretion that can follow major gut resections)
- octreotide (to reduce gastric, biliary and pancreatic secretions)
- antibiotics (if there is small-bowel overgrowth).

Patients with massive resections who are unable to cope on exclusively oral nutrition need referral to specialist centers. They may need regular parenteral supplements of calcium, magnesium, trace elements, essential fatty acids and vitamins, or even total parenteral nutrition administered at home. Rarely, referral for small-bowel transplantation may be required.

TABLE 2.2

Management of short-bowel syndrome

Supportive treatment

- Intravenous fluids and nutrition initially
- Enteral nutrition next
- Small frequent low-fat meals later
- Minimal dietary oxalate
- Specific nutritional supplements as necessary (calcium, magnesium, folate, vitamins, trace elements, essential fatty acids)
- Loperamide, codeine phosphate

Specific measures in severe cases

- Calorie supplementation with medium-chain triglycerides
- Gastric acid inhibition
- Octreotide
- Antibiotics for small-bowel overgrowth
- Home total parenteral nutrition (refer to specialist center)
- Small-bowel transplant (rarely)

Colorectal carcinoma. Patients with chronic extensive ulcerative colitis and Crohn's colitis have an increased risk of colorectal carcinoma; in ulcerative colitis this amounts to a cumulative risk of about 20% after 30 years of disease. Factors increasing the risk of colorectal cancer in both diseases include chronicity of disease, chronically inflamed mucosa, coexistent primary sclerosing cholangitis, a family history of colorectal cancer, adenomatous polyp(s) sited in inflamed mucosa, failure to use aminosalicylate drugs (see Chapter 4) and folate deficiency. In both ulcerative colitis and Crohn's disease, most authorities advocate regular colonoscopic screening with a variety of different methods (see pages 98–100) to detect epithelial dysplasia and/or early cancer, with a view to prompt surgical treatment. However, this approach has not yet been shown unequivocally to reduce mortality from colorectal cancer in IBD.

Small intestinal and anal carcinoma. There is a small but finite risk of these otherwise rare cancers in patients with Crohn's disease: in particular, they occur at sites of very prolonged and severe inflammation.

Extraintestinal associations and complications of IBD

There are many systemic associations and complications of IBD; most affect the liver/biliary tree, joints, skin and eyes (Table 2.3). Most occur in patients with colitis and some largely in those with active disease. In some instances, the condition appears to be a complication of IBD; for example, metabolic complications (gallstones and urinary stones). In others (ankylosing spondylitis, uveitis, arthropathy), there seems to be a genetic and/or immunologic association with IBD. In many cases, the pathogenesis is unknown. Extraintestinal associations and complications with important management implications are outlined below.

Sclerosing cholangitis occurs in about 5% of patients with ulcerative colitis and a smaller proportion of those with Crohn's disease. The pathogenesis is unknown, but the condition may occur years before the onset of overt colitis; 80% of patients have perinuclear antineutrophil cytoplasmic antibodies (pANCAs) in their serum. The condition is characterized by the gradual progression of an inflammatory obliterative fibrosis of the extra- and intrahepatic biliary tree (Figure 2.2), and it is sometimes complicated by cholangiocarcinoma. The risk of colorectal cancer in patients with ulcerative colitis and sclerosing cholangitis exceeds that associated with ulcerative colitis alone.

Patients usually present with complications of biliary stricturing, such as obstructive jaundice, cholangitis or abnormal liver-function tests (raised alkaline phosphatase and γ-glutamyltranspeptidase) at routine screening. The diagnosis may be suggested by ultrasound, computed tomography (CT), magnetic resonance imaging (MRI) and/or liver biopsy; endoscopic retrograde cholangiopancreatography (ERCP) is useful not only for diagnosis (Figure 2.2), but also for the stenting of dominant strictures.

TABLE 2.3

Extraintestinal associations and complications of inflammatory bowel disease

Organ	Complication
Joints/bones	Enteropathic arthropathy*
	Sacroiliitis
	Ankylosing spondylitis
	Clubbing (Crohn's disease only)
	Osteoporosis[†]
Eyes	Episcleritis*
	Uveitis*
Skin	Erythema nodosum*
	Pyoderma gangrenosum
Mouth	Aphthous ulceration
Liver	Fatty change
	Chronic active hepatitis
	Granulomatous hepatitis (Crohn's disease only)
	Cirrhosis
	Amyloid (Crohn's disease only)
Biliary tract	Cholesterol gallstones (terminal ileal Crohn's disease or resection)[†]
	Sclerosing cholangitis
	Cholangiocarcinoma
	Autoimmune pancreatitis
Kidneys	Uric acid stones (total colitis, ileostomy)[†]
	Oxalate stones (terminal ileal Crohn's disease or resection)[†]
Lungs	Fibrosing alveolitis
Blood	Anemia*[†] (iron, B_{12}, folate deficiency)
	Arterial and venous thrombosis[†]
Constitutional	Weight loss*[†]
	Growth retardation (children)*[†]

*Worse when IBD is active.
[†]Complication rather than association.

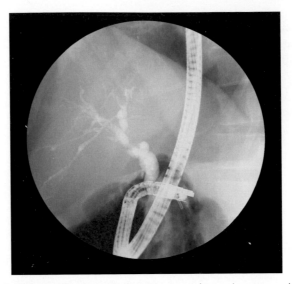

Figure 2.2 Primary sclerosing cholangitis on endoscopic retrograde cholangiopancreatography. Note how the multiple strictures, particularly in the intrahepatic biliary tree, give a beaded appearance.

The course of sclerosing cholangitis is steadily progressive. Oral ursodeoxycholic acid improves pruritus and jaundice. Although it is of unproven benefit in relation to long-term outcome, ursodeoxycholic acid may reduce the incidence of colorectal cancer in those with ulcerative colitis and sclerosing cholangitis. Liver transplant is the only hope of long-term survival in those not developing cholangiocarcinoma; otherwise, median survival for symptomatic patients is about 15 years.

Autoimmune pancreatitis is a recently described rare association with ulcerative colitis. It is characterized by irregular narrowing of the pancreatic duct, and swelling of the gland itself. There are often concomitant biliary changes resembling those found in sclerosing cholangitis. The condition is diagnosed using CT, MRI and/or ERCP; the serum IgG_4 level is also usually raised. The condition responds quickly to prednisolone, but it may recur on withdrawal.

IBD-related arthropathy occurs in up to 10% of patients with IBD. The type of arthritis is determined by human leukocyte antigen (HLA) genotype. IBD-related arthropathy should not be confused with other musculoskeletal pains associated with IBD and its treatment, which include arthralgia related to steroid withdrawal, azathioprine-induced arthralgia and steroid-induced myopathy.

Pauciarticular disease involves fewer than five joints; characteristically, it affects one large joint, for example the knee, and is most common in women. Attacks usually coincide with relapse of colitis; sometimes there is simultaneous erythema nodosum or iritis. Its pathogenesis may involve deposition of gut-derived immune complexes in the affected joint in genetically predisposed individuals. Although the attacks of arthritis may come and go over many years, the disease is neither progressive nor deforming. In most people, the joint symptoms resolve on treatment of the active ulcerative or Crohn's colitis with corticosteroids or, if necessary, surgery. Sulfasalazine may be more effective for the joints than other aminosalicylates. Because aspirin and other NSAIDs may exacerbate IBD (see page 14), they should be avoided if possible. Alternatives include paracetamol (acetaminophen) and joint aspiration with steroid instillation.

Polyarticular IBD-related arthropathy affects more than five joints, particularly small joints such as the metacarpophalangeals. Symptoms are more common in women, are chronic and are not clearly related to activity of the associated IBD. Management resembles that of pauciarticular disease, except that response of the arthropathy to treatment of the IBD itself is poor.

Ankylosing spondylitis. While about 95% of patients without IBD who have ankylosing spondylitis are *HLA-B27*-positive, this is true of only 50–80% of those with both diseases. Ankylosing spondylitis affects about 5% of patients with ulcerative or Crohn's colitis and, like enteropathic arthritis, it is probably immunologically mediated. The patient presents with back pain, stiffness and, in the later stages of the disease, kyphosis (Figure 2.3), diagnosis being confirmed by X-ray. There is often associated sacroiliitis. The course of ankylosing spondylitis is independent of the activity of IBD, and it may present years before the bowel disease becomes manifest. Treatment consists of vigorous physiotherapy, sulfasalazine and, if tolerated, NSAIDs. The

33

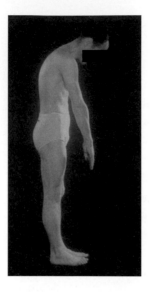

Figure 2.3 Ankylosing spondylitis, showing marked kyphosis. Reproduced courtesy of Dr DP D'Cruz, Guy's, King's and St Thomas' Hospital Medical School, London, UK.

antibody to TNFα, infliximab (see Chapter 4), is an effective therapy in refractory ankylosing spondylitis.

Osteoporosis in IBD is a common consequence of chronic intestinal inflammation, malabsorption and treatment with corticosteroids, particularly a cumulative dose of more than 10 g prednisolone. Its exact prevalence is unclear. The disease is asymptomatic for many years, presenting eventually with vertebral collapse or long bone fractures. To prevent osteoporosis, everyone with IBD should be advised to eat a diet containing adequate calcium and vitamin D, supplemented if necessary by calcium and vitamin D tablets. They should avoid becoming either undernourished or obese (the latter not usually a problem in IBD), stop smoking and take regular exercise.

Those at risk of osteoporosis should undergo bone densitometry. Those with established osteoporosis, or those needing long-term therapy with prednisolone, should receive cyclic bisphosphonate therapy (etidronate). The efficacy of oral budesonide (see Chapter 4) in preventing osteoporosis in steroid-dependent patients with Crohn's disease is not yet proven.

Hormone replacement therapy is associated with an increased risk of breast and gynecologic cancer as well as of thromboembolic disease. Its use in the management of osteoporosis in postmenopausal women should be restricted to those in whom other treatments are ineffective or contraindicated.

Erythema nodosum occurs in about 8% of patients with ulcerative and Crohn's colitis, usually when the disease is active. Hot, red, tender nodules appear, usually on extensor surfaces of the lower legs and arms (Figure 2.4); they gradually subside after a few days to leave brownish skin discoloration. There may be an associated pauciarticular arthropathy. The diagnosis is clinical and biopsy is not necessary. Histology, if performed, shows vasculitis. Treatment is of the active associated IBD.

Pyoderma gangrenosum occurs during the course of IBD in about 2% of patients. There is no clear association with disease activity. Pyoderma presents initially as a discrete pustule with surrounding erythema; this develops into an indolent, painful enlarging ulcer. The most common site is the leg (Figure 2.5). Lesions are occasionally multiple and may occur at sites of recent trauma, for example operation scars. Histology shows lymphocytic vasculitis with dense secondary neutrophilic infiltration. Pyoderma is often refractory to treatment: options include

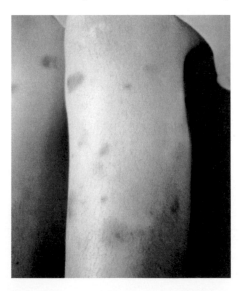

Figure 2.4 Erythema nodosum.

35

Figure 2.5
Pyoderma
gangrenosum:
(a) at presentation;
(b) in the healing
phase.

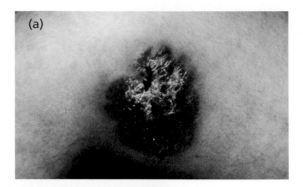

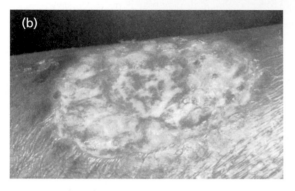

intralesional, topical and systemic corticosteroids, dapsone, heparin and immunosuppressive drugs such as ciclosporin, but the most effective is infliximab. Colectomy does not reliably induce healing of the skin lesion.

Ocular associations. The most common ocular associations of IBD are episcleritis and uveitis. Together they occur in fewer than 5% of patients, usually when the bowel disease is active. Episcleritis presents with burning and itching accompanied by a localized area of dilated blood vessels at the site of scleral inflammation (Figure 2.6). Topical steroids and treatment of the active IBD usually produce a satisfactory response. Uveitis is a more serious and often recurrent problem, presenting with headache, red eye and blurred vision; slit-lamp examination shows pus in the anterior chamber. Treatment includes topical steroids, cycloplegics and therapy of the active IBD. All patients with IBD complicated by ocular symptoms should be promptly referred to an ophthalmologist.

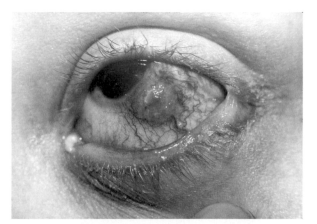

Figure 2.6 Episcleritis in a patient with active ulcerative colitis.

Key points – clinical features and complications

- The presentation of ulcerative colitis depends on its activity and extent, while that of Crohn's disease depends also on the underlying pathological process.
- Intestinal complications of IBD include undernutrition, short-bowel syndrome (in Crohn's disease only) and colorectal cancer.
- The skin, joint, ocular and hepatobiliary associations of IBD are most common in those with colonic disease.
- The course of sclerosing cholangitis and ankylosing spondylitis is unrelated to the activity of the associated IBD.

Key references

Anon. AGA technical review on short bowel syndrome and intestinal transplantation. *Gastroenterology* 2003;124:1111–34.

Bernstein CN, Blanchard JF, Kliewer E et al. Cancer risk in patients with inflammatory bowel disease: a population-based study. *Cancer* 2001;91:854–62.

Bernstein CN, Blanchard JF, Rawsthorne P et al. The prevalence of extraintestinal diseases in inflammatory bowel disease: a population-based study. *Am J Gastroenterol* 2001;96:1116–22.

Krasinskas AM, Raina A, Khalid A et al. Autoimmune pancreatitis. *Gastroenterol Clin North Am* 2007;36:239–57.

Levy C, Lindor KD. Primary sclerosing cholangitis: epidemiology, natural history, and prognosis. *Semin Liver Dis* 2006;26:22–30.

Orchard TR, Thiyagaraja S, Welsh KI et al. Clinical phenotype is related to HLA genotype in the peripheral arthropathies of inflammatory bowel disease. *Gastroenterology* 2000;118: 274–8.

Razack R, Seidner DL. Nutrition in inflammatory bowel disease. *Curr Opin Gastroenterol* 2007;23:400–5.

Silveira M, Lindor K. High dose ursodeoxycholic acid for the treatment of primary sclerosing cholangitis. *J Hepatol* 2008;48: 692–4.

Silverberg MS, Satsangi J, Ahmad T et al. Toward an integrated clinical, molecular and serological classification of inflammatory bowel disease: Report of a Working Party of the 2005 Montreal World Congress of Gastroenterology. *Can J Gastroenterol* 2005;19 (suppl A):5–36.

Soukiasian S, Foster CS, Raizman MB. Treatment strategies for scleritis and uveitis association with inflammatory bowel disease. *Am J Ophthalmol* 1994;118:601–11.

Tung BY, Emond MJ, Haggitt RC et al. Ursodiol use is associated with lower prevalence of colonic neoplasia in patients with ulcerative colitis and primary sclerosing cholangitis. *Ann Intern Med* 2001;134:89–95.

The differential diagnosis of common presentations of IBD is shown in Tables 3.1–3.4. In younger patients (under 50 years) the main differential diagnoses, depending on presentation, include infection and irritable bowel syndrome. In older people (over 50 years), neoplasia, diverticular disease and ischemia require special consideration.

TABLE 3.1

Causes of bloody diarrhea

Cause	Disease
Inflammatory	Ulcerative colitis
	Crohn's colitis
	Behçet's colitis
Infective colitis	Campylobacter
	Salmonella
	Shigella
	Clostridium difficile
	Yersinia
	Tuberculosis
	Enterohemorrhagic *Escherichia coli* (VTEC/0157:H7)
	Amebiasis
	Schistosomiasis
	Cytomegalovirus*
	Herpes simplex*
Neoplastic	Colorectal cancer
Vascular	Ischemia
Iatrogenic	NSAIDs
	Antibiotics
	Irradiation

*Particularly in immunocompromised patients.
NSAIDs, non-steroidal anti-inflammatory drugs.

TABLE 3.2

Causes of rectal bleeding

Cause	Disease
Inflammatory	Proctitis
	Crohn's disease
Sexually transmitted	Gonococcus
	Cytomegalovirus
	Herpes simplex
	Atypical mycobacterium
	Chlamydia
	Kaposi's sarcoma
Neoplasia	Colorectal polyps
	Colorectal cancer
	Anal cancer
Vascular	Ischemia
	Angiodysplasia
Iatrogenic	NSAIDs (oral or suppositories)
	Irradiation
Other	Benign solitary rectal ulcer
	Diverticulosis (acute bleeds only)
	Severe upper gastrointestinal bleeding

NSAIDs, non-steroidal anti-inflammatory drugs.

The aims of investigation (Tables 3.5 and 3.6) are to establish the diagnosis, its site, extent and activity, and to check for complications of the disease and its treatment.

Blood tests

Hematology. In patients presenting with abdominal pain and/or diarrhea, test results revealing anemia, raised platelet count and raised erythrocyte sedimentation rate (ESR) may suggest active IBD, but they are not diagnostic. Those with extensive chronic terminal ileal Crohn's disease may have low serum B_{12}, while a low red-cell folate may indicate active chronic inflammation, reduced intake or malabsorption. Iron deficiency is common, although again it is not diagnostic of IBD.

TABLE 3.3

Causes of abdominal pain, diarrhea and weight loss

Cause	Disease
Inflammatory	Crohn's disease
	Ulcerative colitis
	Microscopic/lymphocytic/collagenous colitis*
	Behçet's colitis
Infections	See Table 3.1
Neoplasia	Colorectal cancer
	Pancreatic cancer
	Small-bowel lymphoma
	Endocrine tumors (carcinoid, gastrinoma, VIPoma)
Endocrine	Thyrotoxicosis
	Diabetic autonomic neuropathy
	Hypoadrenalism
Vascular	Ischemia
Iatrogenic	NSAIDs
	Antibiotics
	Laxative abuse
	Irradiation
	Gut resections
Malabsorption	Celiac disease
	Bacterial overgrowth
	Lactose intolerance†
Other	Irritable bowel syndrome†

*Pain and weight loss unusual. †Weight loss unusual. VIPoma, vasoactive intestinal peptide-producing tumor.

Regular blood counts are necessary to check for bone-marrow depression in patients maintained on immunosuppressive drugs such as azathioprine. Those using sulfasalazine are at risk of hemolytic anemia and folate deficiency as well as bone-marrow depression.

Biochemistry. Raised C-reactive protein and low serum albumin levels suggest active disease in patients with established ulcerative colitis or Crohn's disease; they are also suggestive, although not diagnostic, of

41

TABLE 3.4

Causes of abdominal pain and mass in the right iliac fossa

Cause	Disease
Ileocecal	
Inflammatory	Crohn's disease
	Appendiceal mass
Infective	Tuberculosis
	Ameboma
	Actinomycosis
Neoplastic	Cecal carcinoma
	Lymphoma
	Carcinoid tumor
Other	Fecal loading
Renal	Hydronephrosis
	Cysts
	Neoplasia
	Transplant
Gynecologic	Ovarian cyst
	Neoplasia
	Tubal mass, including ectopic pregnancy
	Endometriosis

IBD in those in whom the diagnosis has not yet been made. Low serum albumin, calcium, magnesium, zinc and essential fatty acid concentrations may be found in Crohn's disease patients with malabsorption, while abnormal liver-function tests may be found in those with hepatobiliary complications of IBD, and require regular monitoring in patients on immunosuppressive therapy.

Serology. In patients presenting for the first time with diarrhea, a negative test for endomysial or transglutaminase antibodies usually excludes celiac disease. Most with ulcerative colitis and a minority with Crohn's disease have circulating perinuclear antineutrophil cytoplasmic antibodies (pANCAs), but this test is not sufficiently sensitive or specific to be of diagnostic value. The diagnostic usefulness of detection

TABLE 3.5

Laboratory investigation of inflammatory bowel disease

Sample	Test
Blood	
Hematology	Hemoglobin
	White blood cells
	Platelets
	Erythrocyte sedimentation rate
	Ferritin
	Vitamin B_{12} (Crohn's disease)
	Red-cell folate
Biochemistry	C-reactive protein
	Liver-function tests
	Albumin
	Calcium, magnesium (suspected malabsorption)
Serology (selected patients)	Endomysial or transglutaminase antibody*
	Amebiasis
	Strongyloidiasis
	Schistosomiasis
	HIV
Stools	Microscopy
	Culture
	Clostridium difficile toxin
	Calprotectin

*To exclude celiac disease. HIV, human immunodeficiency virus.

of circulating antibodies to *Saccharomyces cerevisiae* (ASCA), which are present in most patients with small intestinal Crohn's disease, is also limited. Conceivably, profiles of these and other antibodies, including those against bacterial antigens such as *E. coli* outer membrane porin protein C (OmpC), *Pseudomonas fluorescens* (I2) and flagellin (CBir1), may prove useful in the future in diagnosing patients with IBD of uncertain type.

For patients who have recently traveled to endemic areas, serology (as well as stool samples) should be checked for amebiasis, strongyloidiasis and schistosomiasis. The use of corticosteroids in such

TABLE 3.6

Endoscopy, histopathology and imaging for inflammatory bowel disease

Modality	Test
Endoscopy with biopsy	Sigmoidoscopy (outpatient department)
	Colonoscopy
	Gastroscopy (Crohn's disease, rarely)
	Enteroscopy (Crohn's disease, rarely)
	Wireless capsule endoscopy (Crohn's disease, rarely)
Conventional radiology	Chest X-ray (selected patients)
	Abdominal X-ray
	Barium follow-through or small-bowel enema (Crohn's disease only)
	Fistulography (rarely)
	Barium enema (very rarely)
Isotope scanning	^{99}Tc-HMPAO-labeled leukocyte scan
Other imaging (mainly for Crohn's disease)	Ultrasound (transabdominal and endoscopic)
	CT scan
	MRI

CT, computed tomography; MRI, magnetic resonance imaging; ^{99}Tc-HMPAO, ^{99}technetium hexamethylpropyleneamine oxime.

patients, in the mistaken belief that they have active IBD, can have fatal consequences. HIV testing should be considered for those at risk who have severe diarrhea.

Stool tests

Microscopy. Fresh stools often show red and white blood cells in people with active colitis, whether due to IBD or infection. Hot fresh samples are essential in recent travelers to look for amebic trophozoites.

Culture and toxin assay. Regardless of IBD diagnosis, patients presenting with diarrhea should always have stool samples sent for culture and to check for *Clostridium difficile* toxin. In recent years, as in those without IBD, there has been an increasing incidence of *C. difficile* infection in patients presenting with relapse of their IBD, with a consequent increase in hospitalization rates and deterioration in outcome.

Fecal calprotectin. The transmigration of neutrophils through the mucosa into the lumen is responsible for crypt abscesses and exudate formation. This phenomenon has been exploited to devise an improved marker of disease activity, particularly in Crohn's disease. Fecal levels of calprotectin, a neutrophil-derived cytosolic protein that is resistant to bacterial degradation, provide an accurate index of intestinal inflammatory activity. Although not yet widely used, the test is uncomplicated and promises to be a useful adjunct to routine outpatient clinical assessment.

Sigmoidoscopy and rectal biopsy

Ulcerative colitis. In patients presenting with diarrhea with or without rectal bleeding, rigid or flexible sigmoidoscopy without preparation and without excessive air insufflation can provide immediate confirmation of colitis and its activity (Figure 3.1). Sigmoidoscopy also allows biopsy for histology. To minimize the risks of bleeding and perforation, a small

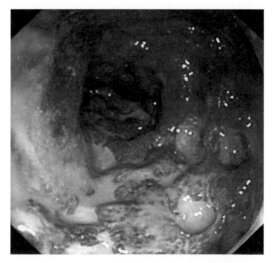

Figure 3.1 Colonoscopic view of acute severe ulcerative colitis, showing deep ulcers with epithelial denudation adjacent to erythematosus edematous mucosa.

superficial biopsy should be taken from the posterior rectal wall less than 100 mm from the anal margin using small-cupped forceps. Rectal biopsy is not routinely necessary for those with established ulcerative colitis. However, in those presenting for the first time, infective colitis as opposed to chronic ulcerative colitis may be suggested by histology showing an acute, focal and superficial infiltrate with minimal goblet-cell depletion and preservation of crypt architecture. Colitis due to C. *difficile*, cytomegalovirus, amebiasis or Crohn's disease sometimes has a characteristic macroscopic appearance, but histology can be used to confirm these diagnoses.

Crohn's disease. Rectal sparing is common in Crohn's colitis. Sometimes, however, rectal induration or ulceration, or the presence of perianal disease, points to the diagnosis. Furthermore, in a minority of patients with macroscopically normal rectal mucosa but Crohn's disease proximal to this site, histology of rectal biopsies shows epithelioid granulomas (see Figure 1.5).

Colonoscopy and biopsy

Ulcerative colitis. In patients who are not severely ill, colonoscopy is the most useful test for confirming the diagnosis of ulcerative colitis and assessing disease extent and activity. It has the advantage over barium enema and radiolabeled leukocyte scanning of allowing biopsies to be taken. Macroscopically, inactive ulcerative colitis is characterized by mucosal edema with loss of the normal vascular pattern, erythema and granularity, while in those with active disease there is, additionally, contact or spontaneous bleeding, excessive mucopus and surface ulceration (see Figure 3.1). In chronic cases, pseudopolyps and loss of the normal haustral pattern with apparent shortening of the colon are common, and in very long-standing disease, the mucosa becomes atrophic.

In patients with acute severe ulcerative colitis, colonoscopy may cause perforation and dilation, and most sick patients can be managed satisfactorily without it. However, colonoscopy plays a major role in cancer surveillance in those with chronic extensive ulcerative colitis (see pages 98–100).

Crohn's disease. Colonoscopy with terminal ileoscopy is central to the macroscopic and microscopic diagnosis of Crohn's disease. It can also be used to balloon-dilate short strictures. In early Crohn's disease, prominent lymphoid follicles (the red-ring sign) are followed by aphthoid ulceration. Later, larger pleomorphic deep ulcers develop, separated by relatively normal-looking mucosa. A cobblestone appearance of the mucosa is a late sign (see Figure 1.4b). Changes in the colon are often segmentally distributed (skip lesions).

Wireless capsule endoscopy. The advent of wireless capsule endoscopy enables non-invasive visualization of small bowel that is inaccessible to the conventional endoscope. The place of this procedure in the investigation of IBD is unclear. It may have a role, for example, in looking for superficial small-bowel mucosal disease suggestive of Crohn's disease (Figure 3.2) in patients with colitis of uncertain type or etiology (CUTE) (see page 23) who have had a normal barium follow-through meal. However, use of this test is compromised by the inability of the capsule, at present, to take biopsies. Furthermore, those with intestinal strictures are at risk of capsule-induced intestinal obstruction.

Radiology
Plain abdominal X-ray
Ulcerative colitis. In patients presenting with active disease, a plain film is useful to assess the extent of disease, since fecal residue on X-ray usually indicates sites of uninflamed colonic mucosa. Plain abdominal radiography is also used to exclude colonic dilation (diameter more than 55 mm) in those with acute severe ulcerative colitis (Figure 3.3). In this setting, severe disease is also indicated by deep ulceration and coarse nodularity of the mucosa, or 'mucosal islands', and linear gas-tracking in the gut wall.

Crohn's disease. A plain film (preferably with the individual both supine and erect) is essential if small-bowel obstruction is suspected. It may also hint at a mass in the right iliac fossa and is helpful, as in ulcerative colitis, in estimating disease extent or severity in active Crohn's colitis. Classically, but exceptionally, complicating radio-opaque urinary stones or gallstones are seen (see Table 2.3; also Chapter 7).

47

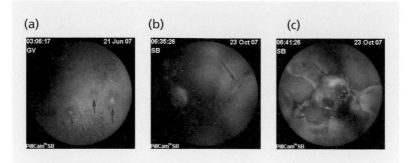

Figure 3.2 Wireless capsule endoscopy images of the small bowel in patients with Crohn's disease: (a) aphthoid ulcers; (b) linear ulcer; (c) more extensive ulceration, mucosal denudation and stricturing. Reproduced courtesy of Dr D Marcos, Barts and The London NHS Trust, London, UK.

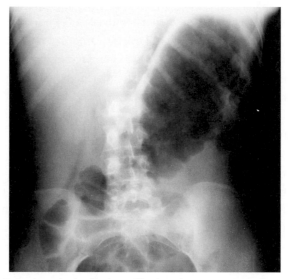

Figure 3.3 Acute colonic dilation affecting the transverse colon.

Contrast and air enemas. Conventional double-contrast barium enema (Figure 3.4) has largely been superseded by colonoscopy. In patients with active colitis, 'air enemas', in which air is gently introduced into the unprepared rectum, are performed in some centers to enhance the information provided by plain abdominal X-ray; in others, 'instant' barium enema is performed without bowel preparation. Neither

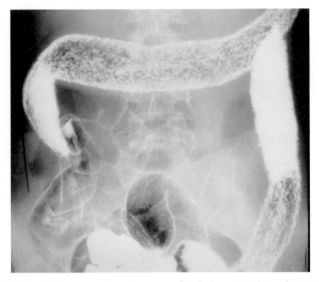

Figure 3.4 Barium enema showing superficial ulceration in active total ulcerative colitis. This test has now been largely superseded by colonoscopy in ulcerative colitis; both tests are potentially dangerous in active disease.

technique, however, adds materially to management in most cases, and both carry a small risk of causing colonic perforation or dilation in severely ill individuals.

Small-bowel radiology. Contrast examination of the small bowel is of central importance in the diagnosis of Crohn's disease proximal to the terminal ileum, showing strictures, ulceration and fistulation (Figure 3.5). Arguments persist about whether conventional barium follow-through or small-bowel enema (enteroclysis) is preferable, but both should be avoided in severely ill patients with Crohn's disease.

Enteroclysis may be more sensitive than barium follow-through for the diagnosis of small lesions and short strictures, but many find the necessary duodenal intubation very uncomfortable. Contrast fistulography is a useful way of clarifying anatomic connections in patients with abdominal sinuses or fistulas.

Radiolabeled leukocyte scans. The intensity and extent of colonic uptake 1 hour after injection of autologous radiolabeled leukocytes

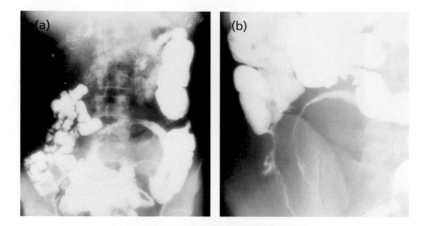

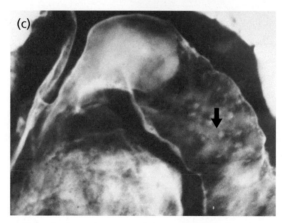

Figure 3.5 Radiological appearance of the small bowel in 3 patients with Crohn's disease: (a) skip lesions causing stricturing at several sites in the ileum; (b) single long terminal ileal stricture; (c) aphthous ulcers (arrowed) in terminal ileum.

provides information, non-invasively, about disease activity, particularly the extent and site, where doubt exists in those with ulcerative colitis or Crohn's disease (Figure 3.6). ^{99}Tc-hexamethylpropyleneamine oxime (^{99}Tc-HMPAO) is preferable to ^{111}indium because of superior definition, lower radiation dose, shorter scanning interval and lower cost. Increased isotopic activity on such scans is not, of course, specific for IBD, since positive results are obtained in other inflammatory gut diseases.

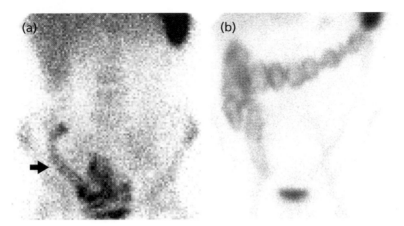

Figure 3.6 Radiolabeled leukocyte scans in 2 patients with Crohn's disease showing inflammation in: (a) the distal ileum (arrowed); (b) the terminal ileum, cecum and ascending and transverse colon.

Delayed scanning can be very helpful in identifying an intra-abdominal abscess, for example in patients with Crohn's disease. In those with mucosal inflammation, delayed scans outline more distal bowel as the radiolabeled leukocytes that have migrated into the lumen move distally. In patients with an abscess, however, the site of uptake remains constant, often gradually intensifying.

Key points – diagnosis

- The aims of investigation are to diagnose IBD, distinguish between ulcerative colitis and Crohn's disease, establish its site, extent and activity, and check for complications of the disease and its treatment.
- Laboratory, endoscopic, histological and imaging tests should be regarded as complementary, but should be undertaken selectively according to individual presentation.
- Clinicians should be aware of the lifetime radiation exposure of individuals with Crohn's and try to avoid inessential use of X-rays and CT scanning.

Ultrasound, CT scanning and MRI. In active Crohn's disease, but not ulcerative colitis, these investigations can be very useful for the evaluation and subsequent percutaneous drainage of localized collections (see Figure 6.5). Computed tomography and MRI will precisely define the anatomy of fistulas and sinuses in Crohn's disease, while all three techniques are now increasingly used for identifying intrinsic gut-wall abnormalities, such as areas of thickening or increased vascularity. Endoluminal ultrasound and MRI (see Figure 6.1) provide the most accurate delineation of perianal abscesses and fistulas.

Increasing awareness of the lifetime radiation exposure of patients with Crohn's disease, together with greater expertise in application, is leading many centers to increase the use of ultrasound and MRI at the expense of contrast radiology and CT scanning.

Key references

Ananthakrishnan AN, McGinley EL, Binion DG. Excess hospitalisation burden associated with *Clostridium difficile* in patients with inflammatory bowel disease. *Gut* 2008;57:205–10.

Gaya DR, Mackenzie JF. Faecal calprotectin: a bright future for assessing disease activity in Crohn's disease. *QJM* 2002;95:557–8.

Giaffer MH. Labelled leucocyte scintigraphy in inflammatory bowel disease: clinical applications. *Gut* 1996;38:1–5.

Iddan G, Meron G, Glukhovsky A et al. Wireless capsule endoscopy. *Nature* 2000;405:417.

Parente F, Maconi G, Bollani S et al. Bowel ultrasound in assessment of Crohn's disease and detection of related small bowel strictures: a prospective comparative study versus x-ray and intraoperative findings. *Gut* 2002;50:490–5.

Scholmerich J. Inflammatory bowel disease. *Endoscopy* 2003;35:164–70.

Silverberg MS, Satsangi J, Ahmad T et al. Toward an integrated clinical, molecular and serological classification of inflammatory bowel disease: Report of a Working Party of the 2005 Montreal World Congress of Gastroenterology. *Can J Gastroenterol* 2005;19 (suppl A):5–36.

Sinha R, Nwokolo C, Murphy PD. Rational imaging. Magnetic resonance imaging in Crohn's disease. *BMJ* 2008;336:273–6.

Stange EF, Travis SPL, Vermeire S et al. European evidence-based consensus on the diagnosis and management of Crohn's disease: definitions and diagnosis. *Gut* 2006;55(suppl 1):1–15.

Drug treatment

This chapter outlines the pharmacology, mechanism of action, indications, side effects, monitoring and contraindications of drugs currently used as specific anti-inflammatory agents in ulcerative colitis and Crohn's disease. Imminent and future developments in medical therapy are also considered.

Corticosteroids

The corticosteroids used in IBD, their indications and their side effects are listed in Table 4.1.

Pharmacology. Corticosteroids can be given intravenously, orally or topically (as a suppository or an enema), the route selected depending on the severity and site of disease. The most widely used oral preparation is prednisolone. Intravenous alternatives are hydrocortisone and methylprednisolone. The former may be marginally more effective in acute severe ulcerative colitis, but it has a greater mineralocorticoid effect. Adrenocorticotropic hormone injections are no longer used: although they are efficacious in those with acute severe ulcerative colitis who have not previously used oral steroids, they offer no practical advantages over conventional corticosteroids.

The systemic side effects of conventional steroids (Table 4.1) have prompted a search for safer formulations. For topical therapy of distal ulcerative colitis, several enema preparations containing steroids that are poorly absorbed and/or undergo rapid first-pass intestinal mucosal and hepatic metabolism are available (e.g. prednisolone metasulfobenzoate and budesonide). These preparations produce fewer systemic side effects and less adrenocortical suppression than hydrocortisone and prednisolone sodium phosphate enemas. A more important advance is the introduction of an oral controlled ileal-release formulation of budesonide for the treatment of active ileocecal Crohn's disease. This drug resembles oral prednisolone in efficacy but, because of its rapid first-pass metabolism, causes much less adrenocortical suppression as

53

TABLE 4.1

Corticosteroids indicated for inflammatory bowel disease

Indications

Active ulcerative colitis and Crohn's disease

Preparations

Intravenous	Hydrocortisone (300–400 mg/day) Methylprednisolone (40–60 mg/day)
Oral	Prednisolone, prednisolone enteric-coated, prednisone (up to 60 mg/day) Budesonide (up to 9 mg/day)
Enemas	Liquid: prednisolone metasulfobenzoate, prednisolone sodium phosphate, budesonide Foam: prednisolone metasulfobenzoate (Predfoam), hydrocortisone (Colifoam)
Suppositories	Hydrocortisone, prednisolone sodium phosphate (Predsol)

Side effects

General	Cushingoid facies, weight gain, dysphoria
Metabolic	Adrenocortical suppression, hyperglycemia, hypokalemia
Cardiovascular	Hypertension, fluid retention
Infection	Intra-abdominal sepsis (Crohn's disease), opportunistic infections, reactivation of tuberculosis, severe chickenpox
Skin	Acne, bruising, striae, hirsuties, delayed wound healing
Eyes	Cataracts, glaucoma
Musculoskeletal	Osteoporosis, avascular osteonecrosis, myopathy
Children	Growth retardation

Monitoring

Blood pressure

Blood sugar/potassium

(CONTINUED)

TABLE 4.1 (CONTINUED)

Contraindications (all relative)	Poorly controlled diabetes or hypertension Osteoporosis Active peptic ulcer Concurrent serious infections

Mechanisms of action

Leukocytes	Reduced migration, activation, survival Reduced activation of NF-κB Phospholipase A2 inhibition Reduced induction of COX-2 and inducible NOS Reduced production of cytokines and lipid mediators Increased kinin degradation
Endothelial cells	Reduced expression of adhesion molecules Reduced capillary permeability

COX, cyclo-oxygenase; NF-κB, nuclear [transcription] factor κB; NOS, nitric oxide synthase.

assessed by plasma cortisol levels. However, it is more expensive than prednisolone. Controlled colonic-release formulations of budesonide and of prednisolone for use in ulcerative and Crohn's colitis are under evaluation.

Mechanism of action. By combining with intracellular glucocorticoid receptors, corticosteroids have many potentially beneficial actions on the inflammatory process (Table 4.1; see also Chapter 1), but which of these is, or are, of predominant importance in IBD is unclear.

Indications. The use of corticosteroids in IBD should be restricted to the treatment of patients with active disease, as there is no evidence that they are able to maintain remission. Corticosteroids continue to have a major role in active ulcerative colitis, but their therapeutic value in Crohn's disease is limited, in part because of their failure to induce mucosal healing. Further details are given in Chapters 5 and 6.

Side effects. The principal side effects of corticosteroids are listed in Table 4.1. They relate to both dose and duration, except for avascular osteonecrosis, which is unpredictable and may occur after only short courses of treatment. In those with fistulating and perianal Crohn's disease, corticosteroids increase the risk of intra-abdominal and pelvic sepsis.

Monitoring treatment. The small minority of patients with IBD who require long-term treatment with oral corticosteroids should have regular checks of their blood pressure and blood sugar and potassium concentrations. Those who exceed a cumulative dose of about 10 g of prednisolone should be assessed for osteoporosis by bone densitometry and treated accordingly (see Chapter 2).

Contraindications. In patients with poorly controlled diabetes mellitus or hypertension, and in those with established osteoporosis or peptic ulceration, alternative pharmacological treatments should be used when possible. As indicated above, steroids should be avoided if possible in those with fistulating Crohn's disease. If steroid therapy is unavoidable, topical therapy or oral budesonide (in those with ileocecal Crohn's disease) is preferable to oral prednisolone.

Aminosalicylates

Pharmacology. 5-Aminosalicylates (5-ASAs) are available in oral formulations (Table 4.2) and as enemas and suppositories (Table 4.3). The original compound, sulfasalazine, consists of 5-aminosalicylic acid linked by an azo bond to sulfapyridine (Figure 4.1; Table 4.2). The sulfonamide moiety acts as a carrier to deliver 5-ASA, the active component, to the colon, where it is released by bacterial action. About 20% of patients cannot tolerate sulfasalazine because of side effects, most of which are due to sulfapyridine (Table 4.3).

The newer oral 5-ASA formulations (Table 4.2) are much better tolerated than sulfasalazine. The pH-dependent, delayed-release and, particularly, slow-release mesalazine preparations also release 5-ASA more proximally in the gut, making them potentially useful in small-bowel Crohn's disease as well as in ulcerative and Crohn's colitis

TABLE 4.2

Representative examples of oral formulations of aminosalicylates (5-ASAs) in inflammatory bowel disease

Drug	Formulation	Dose range (maintenance–conventional maximum)
Prodrugs (5-ASA azo-linked to carrier)		
Sulfasalazine	5-ASA–sulfapyridine	1 g twice daily–2 g three times daily
Olsalazine	5-ASA–5-ASA	500 mg twice daily–1 g three times daily
Balsalazide	5-ASA–aminobenzoylalanine	1.5 g twice daily–2.25 g three times daily
Mesalazine (5-ASA alone) (max. dose 4.8 g daily)		
Delayed-release		
Asacol MR	Eudragit S coating dissolves at pH > 7	400 mg–1.6 g three times daily
Salofalk, Claversal	Eudragit L coating dissolves at pH > 6	500 mg–1 g three times daily
Slow-release		
Pentasa (tablet or sachet)	Ethylcellulose microspheres	500 mg three times daily–2 g twice daily
Salofalk	Granules	500 mg–1 g three times daily
Multimatrix		
Mezavant XL (UK) Lialda (US)	Multimatrix	1.2–4.8 g once daily

Sites to which 5-ASAs are delivered from these formulations are shown in Figure 4.2.

(Figure 4.2). In contrast, olsalazine and balsalazide, like sulfasalazine, release 5-ASA by bacterial azo reduction in the colon and are indicated

TABLE 4.3

Aminosalicylates in inflammatory bowel disease

Indications

Active and inactive ulcerative colitis
Active and inactive Crohn's disease (possibly; see Chapter 6)

Preparations

Oral	See Table 4.2
Enemas	Liquid: Pentasa, Salofalk, sulfasalazine
	Foam: Asacolfoam, Salofalk foam
Suppositories	Asacol, Pentasa, Salofalk, sulfasalazine

Side effects

General	Headache,* fever*
Gut	Nausea,* vomiting,* diarrhea, exacerbation of ulcerative colitis
Blood	Hemolysis,* folate deficiency,* agranulocytosis,* thrombocytopenia,* aplastic anemia,* methemoglobinemia*
Renal	Orange urine,* interstitial nephritis
Skin	Rashes,* toxic epidermal necrolysis,* Stevens–Johnson syndrome,* hair loss
Other	Oligospermia,* acute pancreatitis, hepatitis, lupus syndrome, myocarditis, pulmonary fibrosis

Monitoring

Sulfasalazine	Every 3 months: blood count, red-cell folate, serum urea/creatinine, liver-function tests
Mesalazine	Every 6–12 months: serum urea/creatinine

Contraindications

Sulfasalazine	Known salicylate or sulfonamide sensitivity, G6PDH deficiency, porphyria
Mesalazine	Salicylate sensitivity, renal failure

CONTINUED

TABLE 4.3 (CONTINUED)

Mechanisms of action

Leukocytes	Reduced migration, cytotoxicity
	Reduced activation of NF-κB
	Reduced synthesis of IL-1 and lipid mediators
	Reduced degradation of prostaglandins
	Antioxidant
	TNF antagonist
	Activation of PPAR-γ
Epithelium	Reduced MHC class II expression
	Induction of heat shock proteins
	Reduced apoptosis

*Side effects usually due to sulfonamide component of sulfasalazine.
G6PDH, glucose-6-phosphate dehydrogenase; IL, interleukin; MHC, major histocompatibility complex; NF-κB, nuclear [transcription] factor κB; PPAR-γ, peroxisome proliferator-activated receptor-γ; TNF, tumor necrosis factor.

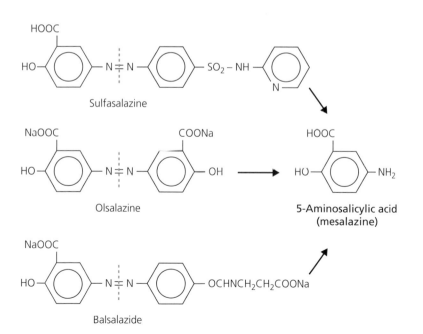

Figure 4.1 Chemistry of 5-aminosalicylate (5-ASA) preparations.

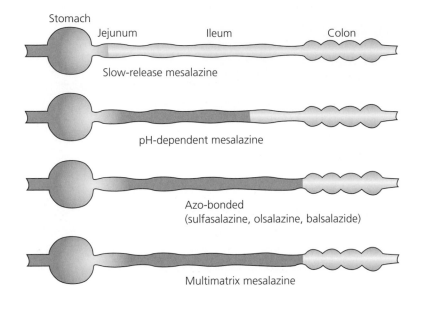

Figure 4.2 Intestinal release profiles of 5-aminosalicylate (5-ASA) formulations (see Table 4.2). There is some variability in the site of release of the various formulations depending on, for example, the precise pH at which 5-ASA is released from different pH-dependent preparations, intestinal intraluminal pH and intestinal transit rate. The multimatrix mesalazine preparation has a pH-dependent coating, while hydrophilic and lipophilic excipients prolong the release of 5-ASA throughout the colon.

for use only in colitis. Very recently, preparations containing higher doses of 5-ASA have become available (800 mg Asacol MR, 1.2 g Mezavant XL/Lialda [UK/US names]), so that patients have to take fewer doses each day. In addition, once-daily administration of Mezavant XL or Pentasa is effective in ulcerative colitis: the increased convenience of once-daily regimens is likely to increase treatment adherence. It is hard to justify not prescribing one of the newer formulations to a patient presenting for the first time with IBD, because of the better tolerability and safety of these preparations. However, in the absence of side effects, those already established on sulfasalazine need not be switched.

Mechanism of action. Like corticosteroids, aminosalicylates have a wide variety of anti-inflammatory effects (see Table 4.3). However, it is not known which of these explains their efficacy in IBD.

Indications and choice of preparation. 5-ASA compounds have a therapeutic role in moderately active (although not acute severe) ulcerative colitis and, particularly, in the prevention of relapse in those with inactive disease. Taken long term, 5-ASA drugs may reduce the risk of development of colorectal cancer in patients with extensive ulcerative colitis. Patients using sulfasalazine in the long term should also be prescribed folic acid to prevent folate deficiency: this may also help to reduce the risk of colonic cancer in chronic extensive ulcerative colitis.

Although mesalazine preparations are moderately effective in active Crohn's disease, the evidence for the usefulness of aminosalicylates in the prevention of symptomatic relapse of quiescent Crohn's disease is equivocal (see Chapter 6).

Side effects. Although better tolerated than sulfasalazine, the newer 5-ASA formulations (see Table 4.2) may cause rash, headache, nausea, diarrhea, exacerbation of ulcerative colitis, pancreatitis and/or blood dyscrasias in up to 5% of patients (see Table 4.3). Interstitial nephritis has been associated very rarely (about 1 in 500 patients) with mesalazine, while watery diarrhea due to active small-intestinal secretion occurs in about 5% of patients given olsalazine. This can usually be avoided by taking the drug with meals.

Monitoring treatment. Patients taking sulfasalazine require regular (every 3–6 months) blood counts, and serum folate and liver-function tests. Those receiving any 5-ASA preparation should have occasional (e.g. annual) checks of their serum urea and creatinine concentrations.

Contraindications. All 5-ASAs should be avoided in those with a history of hypersensitivity to salicylates, including aspirin, or with serious renal impairment. In addition, sulfasalazine should not be given to patients with sulfonamide sensitivity, porphyria or glucose-6-phosphate dehydrogenase deficiency.

Antibiotics

Metronidazole is a nitroimidazole compound with antimicrobial actions against gut anaerobes and protozoa. It also has immunomodulatory effects in vitro. The oral preparation is the most widely used in IBD.

Indications and side effects. Metronidazole, 800 mg/day orally, has moderate benefit in ileocolonic, but not small-bowel, Crohn's disease and in preventing recurrence after ileal resection. Despite the lack of data from controlled trials, it is commonly used in perianal Crohn's disease too. It is also sometimes given in combination with ciprofloxacin in refractory Crohn's disease. Metronidazole has no primary therapeutic role in ulcerative colitis other than in patients with pouchitis following formation of an ileoanal pouch after colectomy (see page 127). Treatment in Crohn's disease must be given for up to 3 months, but it may be confounded by nausea, vomiting, an unpleasant taste in the mouth and/or an individual's unwillingness to abstain from alcohol during this time. The most serious side effect is peripheral neuropathy. This is dose-related, occurs much more often during long-term treatment with 20 mg/kg/day than with 10 mg/kg/day and is not always reversible when treatment ends.

Other antibiotics. Limited data suggest that oral tobramycin and trimethoprim–sulfamethoxazole could improve outcome in acute severe ulcerative colitis. However, most gastroenterologists restrict the use of broad-spectrum antibiotics to prophylaxis against bacteremia and endotoxic shock in severely ill patients with acute severe colitis.

Ciprofloxacin has a moderately beneficial effect in Crohn's disease, particularly in perianal disease; it can also ameliorate pouchitis alone or in combination with metronidazole.

Clarithromycin (sometimes in combination with rifabutin) is reported to have benefit in Crohn's disease and, like metronidazole, has some immunomodulatory effects in vitro.

Antibiotics such as amoxicillin, trimethoprim, ciprofloxacin and metronidazole are sometimes useful for the treatment of diarrhea or steatorrhea due to bacterial overgrowth in patients with small-bowel Crohn's disease, while broad-spectrum and often intravenous antibiotics may be needed, together with drainage, in the management of those with intra-abdominal or perianal abscesses complicating Crohn's disease.

Probiotics and prebiotics

Probiotics are defined as live microorganisms which, when given orally in sufficient quantity, confer a health benefit on the host. Given the importance of intestinal bacterial flora in driving the mucosal inflammation characteristic of IBD, it is unsurprising that a range of probiotic organisms have been assessed for its treatment (listed later in Table 4.7). To date, evidence of efficacy relates only to use of *E. coli* Nissle to prevent relapse of ulcerative colitis, and of VSL3, which contains a mixture of bifidobacteria, lactobacilli and streptococci, in pouchitis.

Prebiotics are non-digestible food ingredients, particularly certain sugars, that beneficially affect the host by selectively stimulating the growth of probiotic bacteria in the gut. Trials are under way to assess their therapeutic efficacy as food supplements in IBD.

Nothwithstanding the paucity of data confirming the benefits of probiotics and prebiotics in IBD, they are widely used by patients adopting a complementary or alternative medical approach to their illness (see page 77): they are, at least, probably safe.

Immunomodulatory drugs

Immunomodulatory agents currently used in the treatment of IBD include azathioprine and its active metabolite mercaptopurine (MP) and, less often, ciclosporin and methotrexate.

Azathioprine and mercaptopurine. Azathioprine is a prodrug that undergoes rapid conversion to MP; both are imidazole purine analogs (thiopurines). The doses most commonly used in IBD are 2.0 and 1.0 mg/kg/day, respectively (Table 4.4). Both drugs are currently used only in oral formulations and take up to 4 months to exert their clinical benefit. Intravenous azathioprine does not, unfortunately, accelerate the response in active IBD.

Homozygous deficiency of thiopurine methyltransferase (TPMT), an enzyme responsible for the safe metabolism of azathioprine and MP,

TABLE 4.4

Azathioprine and mercaptopurine (MP) in inflammatory bowel disease

Indications

Steroid-dependent or -refractory ulcerative colitis and Crohn's disease

Fistulating and perianal Crohn's disease

Preparations

Oral	Azathioprine (2.0–2.5 mg/kg/day)
	MP (1.0–1.5 mg/kg/day)

Side effects

General	Nausea, vomiting, headache, arthralgia, fever, rash, abdominal pain
Blood	Agranulocytosis, thrombocytopenia, macrocytosis
Infections	Opportunistic including cytomegalovirus, herpes zoster
Hepatobiliary	Cholestatic hepatitis, acute pancreatitis
Malignancy	Lymphoma, skin (possibly)

Monitoring

Blood count, liver-function tests

Every 2 weeks for the first 2 months, then every 2–3 months

Contraindications

Pregnancy (relative contraindication)

Thiopurine methyltransferase (TPMT) deficiency

Concurrent allopurinol

Mechanism of action

Inhibition of T-cell DNA synthesis

occurs in about 0.2% of the population. This enzyme deficiency is likely to account for some of the serious untoward effects that can occur with thiopurines. In many centers, TPMT assay is now undertaken before thiopurine treatment is initiated, primarily to reduce the chance of severe thiopurine-induced bone-marrow suppression in those with homozygous enzyme deficiency.

Mechanism of action. The precise mechanism of action of azathioprine and MP is not known, but they appear to modify the immune response by inhibiting DNA synthesis in T cells. Azathioprine has anti-inflammatory and antibacterial as well as immunomodulatory effects.

Indications. Azathioprine and MP are used predominantly as steroid-sparing agents in those with steroid-dependent or steroid-refractory IBD. They may also have special roles in accelerating remission and healing ileal lesions when given in combination with prednisolone in active Crohn's disease and in fistulating Crohn's disease, particularly perianal disease.

Side effects. Up to 20% of patients cannot tolerate azathioprine because of its side effects (see Table 4.4). A switch to MP may avert these problems in about half. More seriously, both drugs cause acute pancreatitis in about 3% of people. Other potentially serious side effects of dose-dependent bone-marrow depression (particularly in the first few weeks of treatment: 2% of patients) and cholestatic hepatitis necessitate regular blood monitoring. There is an increased risk of infections, particularly a serious form of glandular fever. Very long-term use, as in transplant patients, may yet prove to increase the risk of malignancy, including lymphoma. Indeed, white patients taking azathioprine or MP should avoid excessive exposure to sunlight because of the risk of skin cancer.

Monitoring treatment. Patients started on azathioprine or MP should have blood counts every 2 weeks for the first 2 months of therapy to check for incipient bone-marrow depression. Thereafter, white-cell count, platelet count and liver-function tests should be performed every 2–3 months.

Contraindications. Several series have allayed previous fears about the safety of thiopurines in pregnancy (see Chapter 8): flare of disease activity induced by stopping azathioprine or MP in pregnancy is likely to be more dangerous to the fetus than continuing with these drugs. Patients receiving allopurinol should not be given either drug because the allopurinol inhibits xanthine oxidase, thus reducing metabolism of azathioprine and MP.

Methotrexate acts predominantly by inhibiting the enzymes that metabolize folic acid. At high doses, the main enzyme affected is dihydrofolate reductase, with consequent inhibition of RNA, DNA and protein synthesis. At the lower doses used to treat Crohn's disease, the anti-inflammatory and immunomodulatory effects of methotrexate are likely to result from inhibition of other folate-dependent enzymes.

Indications. Given once weekly as a 25-mg intramuscular injection, methotrexate improves symptoms and reduces steroid requirements in chronically active steroid-dependent Crohn's disease. An intramuscular dose of 15 mg/week maintains remission in such patients. Most gastroenterologists resort first to a thiopurine rather than to methotrexate in steroid-resistant or steroid-dependent patients with Crohn's disease; many prescribe it orally rather than by injection. Although not yet proven to be effective in ulcerative colitis in formal clinical trials, methotrexate is used in many centers for patients with colitis who have been intolerant of or refractory to thiopurines.

Side effects necessitate discontinuation of methotrexate in up to 20% of people. Nausea, vomiting, stomatitis and diarrhea are the most common. As with other immunosuppressive agents, there is an increase in opportunistic infections and bone-marrow depression. These side effects are reduced by coadministration of folic acid, which does not compromise the therapeutic effectiveness of methotrexate. Hepatic fibrosis and pneumonitis are the most serious side effects of long-term therapy with methotrexate in patients with psoriasis and rheumatoid arthritis, but they appear to be less common in those with IBD.

Monitoring treatment. The risk of bone-marrow depression necessitates weekly blood counts for the first 4 weeks, and thereafter every 1–2 months. Folic acid should also be coadministered at a dose of 1–5 mg/day.

Liver-function tests, including albumin, should be monitored every 1–2 months. Liver biopsy is probably unnecessary, except in those with persistently abnormal liver-function tests or after a cumulative dose of more than 5 g.

Unexplained shortness of breath or coughing necessitates a chest X-ray and blood gas and lung-function tests, particularly measurement of carbon monoxide diffusing capacity.

Contraindications. Pregnancy and conception should be avoided within 6 months of the treatment of either partner, because methotrexate is teratogenic. Breastfeeding is also contraindicated. Coadministration of other antifolate agents, such as trimethoprim–sulfamethoxazole, may increase the toxic effects of methotrexate on the bone marrow, as may NSAIDs, penicillin, old age and renal impairment.

To reduce the risk of hepatotoxicity, methotrexate should not be prescribed to patients who drink more than seven units of alcohol per week, weigh over 40% more than their recommended weight for height, or have diabetes mellitus.

Ciclosporin is a fungus-derived cyclic undecapeptide useful in steroid-refractory severe active ulcerative colitis. Intravenous therapy is usually given initially, being replaced after a few days with the oral preparation (Neoral). Recent reports suggest that a lower dose of 2 mg/kg/day (intravenous) is as effective as, and safer than, the initially recommended dose of 4 mg/kg/day (intravenous). Close monitoring of whole blood concentrations is used to adjust ciclosporin dosage. The target levels depend on the method used for analysis and on the route of administration (Table 4.5). Because ciclosporin is metabolized via the cytochrome P450 enzyme system, grapefruit juice and drugs that inhibit this enzyme system should be taken with caution. However, drugs that induce the cytochrome P450 system decrease blood levels of ciclosporin (Table 4.5).

Mechanism of action. Ciclosporin reduces helper and cytotoxic T-cell function and proliferation by inhibiting IL-2 gene transcription.

Indications. Initial enthusiasm for intravenous ciclosporin in active Crohn's disease and ciclosporin enemas in distal ulcerative colitis was not justified by later reports. The only current indication for ciclosporin in IBD is as an adjunctive treatment in steroid-refractory acute severe ulcerative colitis (see Chapter 5).

TABLE 4.5

Ciclosporin in inflammatory bowel disease

Indications

Steroid-refractory acute severe ulcerative colitis (intravenous then oral)

Preparations

Oral	Neoral, 5 mg/kg/day
Intravenous	2–4 mg/kg/day by continuous infusion

Side effects

General	Nausea, vomiting, headache
Renal	Interstitial nephritis
Infection	Opportunistic, including *Pneumocystis carinii* pneumonia
Neurological	Epileptic fits, paresthesias, myopathy
Cardiovascular	Hypertension
Skin	Hypertrichosis, gingival hypertrophy
Metabolic	Hyperkalemia, hypomagnesemia, hyperuricemia
Liver	Cholestatic hepatitis
Malignancy	Lymphoma

Monitoring

Pre-treatment	Serum urea and creatinine, potassium, magnesium, cholesterol, urate, liver function
On treatment	Aim for blood ciclosporin concentrations: • 250–400 ng/mL for intravenous • trough 150–300 ng/mL for oral Serum urea and creatinine, potassium, magnesium, urate, liver function Blood pressure

Contraindications

Pregnancy, lactation	Renal impairment, hypertension, infection, epilepsy, malignancy

CONTINUED

TABLE 4.5 (CONTINUED)	
Disease	Low serum cholesterol or magnesium, high potassium
Biochemical	Coadministration of cytochrome P450 inhibitors (grapefruit juice, erythromycin, oral contraceptives, fluconazole, calcium-channel and proton-pump inhibitors)
Drugs	Coadministration of cytochrome P450 inducers (phenytoin, barbiturates, rifampicin, carbamazepine)

Mechanism of action

Inhibition of IL-2 gene transcription leading to inhibition of helper and cytotoxic T-cell function and proliferation

IL-2, interleukin-2.

Side effects and monitoring. The most serious side effects of ciclosporin are:

- opportunistic infections (occurring in 20% of patients), such as *Pneumocystis carinii* pneumonia, for which coadministration of prophylactic trimethoprim–sulfamethoxazole may be advisable
- renal impairment, including a 20% reduction in glomerular filtration rate in most patients and, in 25%, an interstitial nephritis that is not always reversible when treatment stops
- hypertension (30% of patients)
- hepatotoxicity (up to 20% of patients)
- epileptic fits (3% of patients) due to penetration of the blood–brain barrier by Cremophor, a lipid-soluble vehicle for intravenous ciclosporin; the fits are confined to those with low serum cholesterol and/or magnesium concentrations, and do not occur with oral ciclosporin.

Long-term oral use of ciclosporin, for which there is no clear indication in IBD, may predispose to lymphoma. The side effects of the drug will prevent it ever becoming widely used for IBD. Its use demands frequent monitoring of ciclosporin blood levels and serum biochemistry.

Tacrolimus is another oral macrolide immunosuppressant derived originally from a bacterium and widely used in transplant medicine. Its side effects, which mostly resemble those of ciclosporin, include induction of diabetes mellitus. Use of tacrolimus requires careful monitoring of drug levels, blood sugar and renal function. In IBD, the drug is restricted to those with very refractory disease.

Modulation of cytokine activity

Our increased understanding in recent years of the etiopathogenesis of IBD (see Chapter 1) has prompted trials using a wide range of antibodies and other agents specifically targeting abnormal cytokine expression (listed later in Table 4.7). Of these, only antibodies against tumor necrosis factor α (TNFα) have so far reached routine clinical use. In the long term, it is likely that a range of other cytokine-based therapies will enter clinical practice, at least for those with refractory IBD. These may include gene transfer techniques to induce intestinal mucosal production of anti-inflammatory cytokines, such as IL-4 and IL-10.

Anti-TNFα antibodies. Infliximab (Remicade), a mouse–human chimeric anti-TNFα antibody, was launched for the treatment of Crohn's disease in the USA in 1998 and in the UK and Europe in 1999. The use of antibodies has revolutionized the management of other chronic inflammatory diseases such as rheumatoid arthritis, and has proven a major advance for patients with refractory or fistulous Crohn's disease and, to a lesser extent, ulcerative colitis. Adalimumab (Humira), which has been introduced more recently, is a fully humanized anti-TNFα antibody. At present, it is used mainly for those losing response to, or intolerant of, infliximab, since these problems are usually due to formation of antibodies to the murine component of infliximab (antibodies to infliximab, ATI) which is not present in adalimumab. In the US and some other countries, a third anti-TNFα antibody, certolizumab pegol (Cimzia), is also licensed for use in Crohn's disease. Reassurance is still needed that the clear therapeutic benefits produced by these drugs will not, in the very long term, be outweighed by serious adverse effects, in particular infection and/or malignancy. In the future, it is possible that anti-TNFα antibodies will be replaced by non-protein small-molecule drugs that prevent the production or actions of TNF: an existing example is thalidomide, the possible benefits of which are confounded by its side effects, especially in relation to pregnancy.

Pharmacology. Infliximab is usually administered using an induction regimen of infusions at 0, 2 and 6 weeks, followed by regular infusions at intervals of 8 weeks, each infusion being given over 1–2 hours. The standard dose is 5 mg/kg per infusion, and the cost is about $2400/£1200/€2000 per infusion. Some patients losing response need 10 mg/kg, or more frequent infusions. In acute severe steroid-refractory ulcerative colitis, a single infusion of 5 mg/kg halves the risk of colectomy (see Chapter 5).

Adalimumab, in contrast to infliximab, is given by subcutaneous infusion. Induction is usually with doses of 80 and 40 mg at an interval of 2 weeks; subsequent injections of 40 mg are given every other week, although many patients losing their initial response need to increase to 40 mg every week. At standard doses, adalimumab is slightly cheaper than infliximab.

Certolizumab pegol, which is a pegylated humanized anti-TNFα antibody, is given subcutaneously as a 400 mg dose at 0, 2 and 4 weeks, then every 4 weeks.

Mechanism of action. The antibodies appear to act by binding not only to free TNFα but also to surface-bound TNFα on activated T cells, leading to their apoptosis. The net result is downregulation of the cytokine cascade (see Chapter 1).

Indications. Intravenous infusions of infliximab often induce remission in active and otherwise refractory Crohn's disease, and heal perianal and other fistulas in Crohn's disease (see Chapter 6). In general, 30% of patients with previously refractory Crohn's disease achieve remission, 30% improve substantially while the rest do not improve. As indicated above, adalimumab and certolizumab pegol are usually reserved for those losing their response to, or who are intolerant of, infliximab. Infliximab is of moderate efficacy in refractory outpatient ulcerative colitis, and halves the colectomy rate in inpatients with steroid-refractory acute severe colitis; however, its role is less clear in these settings than in Crohn's disease in view of the conventional alternative option of surgery (see Chapter 5). Anti-TNFα antibody is useful in minimizing steroid usage and in preventing growth retardation in children with active Crohn's disease, but concerns about its safety necessitate particularly careful control of its use in this group.

The effects of infliximab in adults with severe complicated Crohn's disease are impressive, mucosal lesions sometimes healing completely. Co-prescription of azathioprine, MP or methotrexate appears to prolong the response to infliximab, possibly by reducing the development of ATI and subsequent hypersensitivity reactions. Such concurrent immunosuppression may, however, increase the risks of opportunistic infection and lymphoma, so that many gastroenterologists recommend discontinuation of thiopurines or methotrexate after 6 months of treatment with infliximab. In the future, the selection of patients for treatment with anti-TNFα antibody may depend not only on their disease phenotype (e.g. fistulating disease), but also on their genotype. For example, some evidence suggests that patients with Crohn's disease who are positive for pANCA and have particular TNFα microsatellite haplotypes show a poor response to infliximab.

Side effects. Common side effects associated with the infusion of infliximab include headache, rash, nausea and fever (Table 4.6). These are usually mild and respond to antihistamines. However, anaphylaxis may occur, so antihistamines, adrenaline and corticosteroids should be on hand when infusions are given. Repeat infusions of infliximab after an interval of more than 20 weeks increase the risk of developing ATI: these may reduce the efficacy of infliximab and can cause a delayed serum-sickness-like reaction, characterized by myalgia, arthralgia, rash and fever. This reaction responds to prednisolone and analgesics, but may contraindicate further treatment. Intravenous hydrocortisone given prior to infliximab may reduce the formation of ATI. Adalimumab injections are often painful.

Several infections have been described in patients receiving anti-TNFα antibodies, the most serious being tuberculosis (TB). When it occurs, TB is disseminated in over 50% of cases and extrapulmonary in about 25%. To date, it has caused more than 100 deaths worldwide. Anti-TNFα antibodies can also exacerbate congestive cardiac failure.

TABLE 4.6

Anti-TNFα antibodies, infliximab, adalimumab and certolizumab pegol in inflammatory bowel disease

Indications

Steroid-dependent or -refractory active Crohn's disease
Fistulating Crohn's disease
Steroid-dependent/-refractory ulcerative colitis (in some countries)
Pyoderma gangrenosum
Ankylosing spondylitis

Preparations	
Intravenous	Infliximab (Remicade), 5–10 mg/kg per infusion
Subcutaneous	Adalimumab (Humira), 40 mg every other week or weekly (after 80 mg initial dose)
	Certolizumab pegol (Cimzia), 400 mg every 4 weeks

Side effects	
General	Headache (20%), nausea (10%), upper respiratory tract infection (10%)
Serious infections	Tuberculosis, salmonella, cellulitis, pneumonia
Infusion reactions	Headache, rash, nausea, fever
Intestinal	Obstruction
Autoantibodies	Infliximab only: ATI (delayed hypersensitivity) Antibodies to DNA and cardiolipin (lupus syndrome)
Malignancy	Lymphoma including hepatosplenic T-cell lymphoma in young patients also on azathioprine
Neurological	Aseptic meningitis, demyelination
Cardiac	Congestive cardiac failure

Monitoring

Check TB history

Chest X-ray

PPD skin test (Mantoux) or Quantiferon test (some countries)

CONTINUED

TABLE 4.6 (CONTINUED)

During and 1 hour after infusions:

- pulse
- blood pressure
- respiration
- temperature

Contraindications

Pregnancy (current or planned in next 6 months – see text), lactation

Active infection

Current or previous malignancy

Tight strictures or obstructive symptoms

Previous TB, multiple sclerosis, heart failure

Hypersensitivity to murine proteins

Mechanism of action

Binding of surface-bound T-cell TNF and free TNF

ATI, antibodies to infliximab; PPD, purified protein derivatives; TB, tuberculosis; TNF, tumor necrosis factor.

Possible neurological complications include aseptic meningitis and irreversible demyelination. In patients with pre-existing intestinal strictures, rapid healing by fibrosis has been reported occasionally to precipitate bowel obstruction.

There are isolated reports of lymphoma in those receiving anti-TNFα antibodies for Crohn's disease or rheumatoid arthritis. Hepatosplenic T-cell lymphoma is an extremely rare but almost invariably lethal complication which appears mainly in young patients with Crohn's concurrently treated with infliximab or adalimumab and a thiopurine.

Although formally contraindicated in pregnancy, the outcome of unintended pregnancies in women receiving infliximab for rheumatoid arthritis and IBD has been reassuring. Antibodies to double-stranded DNA and to cardiolipin have been observed in up to 15% of patients who receive infliximab for Crohn's disease, and a transient lupus syndrome has been reported in those with rheumatoid arthritis.

Contraindications to the use of anti-TNFα antibodies are shown in Table 4.6. Most of these relate to the potential side effects of treatment described above.

Monitoring. To minimize the risk of reactivated, disseminated TB, patients should have a careful history for previous TB and a chest X-ray before infusion of anti-TNFα antibodies; in most countries a PPD (Mantoux) skin or Quantiferon test is also recommended. Pulse, blood pressure, respiratory rate and temperature measurements should also be taken half-hourly during, and for 1 hour after, treatment to minimize the risk of infusion reactions. Infusions should be carried out in hospitals with full resuscitation facilities available, but they may be performed on an outpatient basis.

New therapeutic approaches

Progressive elucidation of the pathogenesis of IBD (Chapter 1) has led to the evaluation, in experimental animal models of IBD and to a lesser extent in humans, of a number of further therapeutic approaches aimed at specific pathophysiological targets (Figure 4.3, Table 4.7). Over the next few years, several of these options are likely to reach the bedside, particularly for patients with disease refractory to current treatments.

TABLE 4.7

Potential new treatments for inflammatory bowel disease aimed at specific pathophysiological targets

Target	Agent
Colonic flora	Probiotics (bifidobacteria, *Lactobacillus* spp., non-pathogenic *E. coli* including *E. coli* Nissle)* Prebiotics Porcine whipworm (*Trichuris suis*) eggs
Mucus layer and epithelium	Phosphatidylcholine Short-chain fatty acid enemas,* epidermal growth factor enemas Trefoil peptides Growth hormone

CONTINUED

75

TABLE 4.7 (CONTINUED)

Leukocytes

Reduce or increase numbers	Apheresis (Adacolumn, Cellsorba)*, stem-cell transplant*, granulocyte colony-stimulating factor
Reduce migration	Adhesion-molecule antibodies (nataluzimab, MLN02), antisense oligonucleotides (ICAM-1)
T-cell blockade	Anti-CD3 (visilizumab)*, anti-CD25 (basiliximab, daclizumab)*, costimulatory blockade (abatacept)*
Modify intra-cellular signaling	PPAR-γ agonist (rosiglitazone), MAP kinase inhibitor signaling

Cytokines

Reduce proinflammatory cytokines	NF-κB antisense oligonucleotide
Antagonize inflammatory cytokines	Anti-interferon-γ (fontolizumab)*, anti-IL-12/23 antibodies, IL-1 receptor antagonist
Increase anti-inflammatory cytokines	IL-10, interferon-α or -β, IL-11, TGF-β, IL-4 gene therapy

Mediators	Cytoprotective prostaglandins, COX-2 inhibition
	Synthesis inhibitors and receptor antagonists of leukotrienes, thromboxanes
	Antioxidants
	Inducible NOS inhibition
	Fish oil (eicosapentenoic acid [EPA])
	Metalloproteinase inhibitors
Enteric nerves	Local anesthetics (lidocaine, ropivercaine enemas)*

Unknown targets	Nicotine (ulcerative colitis)*, stopping smoking (Crohn's disease)*

*Current or imminent option. COX, cyclo-oxygenase; ICAM-1, intercellular adhesion molecule; IL, interleukin; MAP, mitogen-activated protein; NF-κB, nuclear [transcription] factor κB; NOS, nitric oxide synthase; PPAR-γ, peroxisome proliferator-activated receptor-γ; TGF, transforming growth factor.

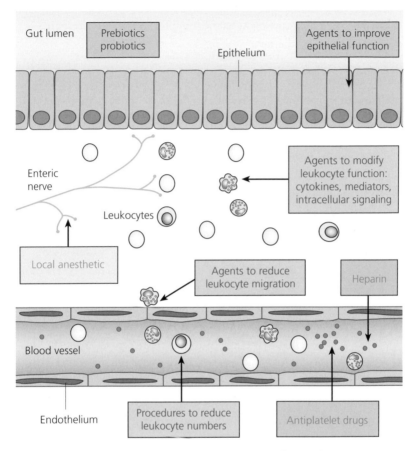

Figure 4.3 The specific pathophysiological targets of new therapeutic approaches.

Complementary and alternative therapy

The terms 'complementary' and 'alternative' medicine denote theories and practices in medicine that deviate from conventional ones. The former applies to adjunctive therapies, while the latter applies to treatments that are used instead of standard management. The combined term comprises a heterogeneous range of diagnostic and therapeutic procedures, ranging from traditional practices such as acupuncture, traditional Chinese medicine, homeopathy and herbal medicine, to more modern complementary practices such as aromatherapy and reflexology. Indeed, we suggest that the term 'comprehensive' therapy might be more appropriate than 'alternative' or 'complementary' therapy.

Current usage. Recent surveys have shown that up to 50% of people in the Western world use complementary therapies. Indeed, approximately half of patients with gastrointestinal disorders, including IBD, have used complementary therapies, most commonly herbal remedies. The widespread use of such therapies in IBD is likely to be related to the chronic and refractory nature of the disease, and has been linked with poor quality of life in terms of psychosocial functioning.

Effectiveness. Limited data suggest that aloe vera, *Boswellia serrata*, wheat grass juice, curcumin (the yellow pigment of the widely used spice, turmeric) and some traditional Chinese medicines may be effective in ulcerative colitis. In addition, acupuncture appears to benefit some with IBD. Despite the difficulties in evaluating complementary medicine, in view of the widespread use of complementary approaches by patients with IBD, it is essential that efforts are made to assess scientifically the effectiveness and safety of, at least, the most frequently used therapies.

Side effects. While it is unlikely that therapies such as reflexology will have direct adverse effects, the same cannot be said of herbal therapies: adverse effects have included fatal liver toxicity as well as irreversible renal failure. The interaction of herbal therapies with conventional drugs needs further clarification. In the context of IBD, however, St John's wort reduces blood levels of ciclosporin by enhancing the activity of cytochrome P450 enzymes, while gingko, ginger and devil's claw reduce the absorption of orally administered iron.

Perhaps more importantly, complementary and alternative therapies may be associated with indirect adverse effects. For example, patients who initially consult an alternative practitioner may suffer from misdiagnosis, while others may delay or forego appropriate conventional options in favor of ineffective unconventional ones.

There is an urgent need for further scientific assessment of the benefits and dangers of complementary therapies. Herbal preparations, in particular, should require licensing by an independent national body in order to improve their quality and safety, while claims of effect should be validated by controlled trials. The general public, pharmacists and doctors need to be aware of the direct and indirect risks associated with the use of complementary therapies.

Key points – drug treatment

- Treatment for IBD has improved substantially, owing to new formulations and better use of conventional drugs, including corticosteroids, aminosalicylates, antibiotics and immunomodulatory agents.
- Anti-TNFα antibodies (infliximab, adalimumab and certolizumab pegol) represent an important advance for patients with refractory or fistulous Crohn's disease; infliximab can also be helpful in refractory active ulcerative colitis. The possibility of serious side effects, including infection and malignancy, needs to be borne in mind for all patients on these treatments.
- Treatment of IBD is likely to improve further with the advent of new biological therapies arising from improved understanding of the pathogenesis of the disease.
- Complementary and alternative therapies are widely used for IBD, but there are insufficient data on their effectiveness and safety.

Key references

D'Haens G. Risks and benefits of biologic therapy for inflammatory bowel diseases. *Gut* 2007;56: 725–32.

Faubion WA Jr, Loftus EV Jr, Harmsen WS et al. The natural history of corticosteroid therapy for inflammatory bowel disease: a population-based study. *Gastroenterology* 2001;121:255–60.

Feagan BG, Rochon J, Fedorak RN et al. Methotrexate for the treatment of Crohn's disease. The North American Crohn's Study Group Investigators. *N Engl J Med* 1995;332:292–7.

Greenberg GR, Feagan BG, Martin F et al. Oral budesonide for active Crohn's disease. *N Engl J Med* 1994; 331:836–41.

Hanauer SB, Feagan BG, Lichtenstein GR et al. Maintenance infliximab for Crohn's disease: the ACCENT 1 randomised trial. *Lancet* 2002;359: 1541–9.

Irving PM, Shanahan F, Rampton DS. Drug interactions in inflammatory bowel disease. *Am J Gastroenterol* 2008;103:207–19.

Järnerot G, Hertervig E, Friis-Liby I et al. Infliximab as rescue therapy in severe to moderately severe ulcerative colitis: a randomized, placebo-controlled study. *Gastroenterology* 2005;128:1805–11.

Kamm MA, Sandborn WJ, Gassull M et al. Once-daily, high-concentration MMX mesalamine in active ulcerative colitis. *Gastroenterology* 2007;132:66–75.

Langmead L, Rampton DS. Review article: complementary and alternative therapies for inflammatory bowel disease. *Aliment Pharmacol Ther* 2006;23:341–9.

Lichtiger S, Present DH, Kornbluth A et al. Cyclosporine in severe ulcerative colitis refractory to steroid therapy. *N Engl J Med* 1994;330:1841–5.

Pearson DC, May GR, Fick GH et al. Azathioprine and 6-mercaptopurine in Crohn's disease: a meta-analysis. *Ann Intern Med* 1995;122:132–42.

Peyrin-Biroulet L, Desreumaux P, Sandborn WJ, Colombel JS. Crohn's disease: beyond antagonists of tumour necrosis factor. *Lancet* 2008;372: 67–81.

Present DH, Rutgeerts P, Targan S et al. Infliximab for the treatment of fistulas in patients with Crohn's disease. *N Engl J Med* 1999; 340:1398–405.

Rutgeerts P, Sandborn WJ, Feagan BG et al. Infliximab for induction and maintenance therapy for ulcerative colitis. *N Engl J Med* 2005;353:2462–76.

Sandborn WJ, Rutgeerts P, Enns R et al. Adalimumab induction therapy for Crohn disease previously treated with infliximab: a randomized trial. *Ann Intern Med* 2007;146:829–38.

Shanahan F. Inflammatory bowel disease: immunodiagnostics, immunotherapeutics, and ecotherapeutics. *Gastroenterology* 2001;120:622–35.

The management of patients with ulcerative colitis, as for Crohn's disease, comprises general measures, supportive treatment and specific pharmacological and surgical therapies. The aims of treatment are to induce and then maintain remission.

General measures

The general principles of management of IBD are summarized in Table 5.1.

Explanation and psychosocial support. Patients with newly diagnosed ulcerative colitis need a full explanation from their doctor and/or specialist IBD nurse about their disease and its implications. All patients with IBD need to be given advice as to how best to help themselves; some suggestions are shown in Table 5.2.

The process of learning about IBD can be facilitated by the written information and other services provided by patient support groups (for a list of addresses, see the section at the back of this book entitled 'Useful resources').

The services offered by such groups include:
• educational literature, websites and helplines
• lecture and discussion meetings at which patients and their families can share their problems
• specialist counseling for individuals with particular difficulties relating to their illness.
These groups can also provide direction to the appropriate social agencies to help with employment problems, and to insurance companies for life, travel and motor insurance.

Lastly, large patient support groups can act as a political pressure group to help maximize accessibility of healthcare services to patients with both kinds of IBD, and play a major role in generating funds for research.

TABLE 5.1

Principles of the management of inflammatory bowel disease

General measures

Explanation, psychosocial support

- physicians, specialist nurses
- patient support groups

Specialist multidisciplinary hospital care

- monitoring disease activity, nutrition, therapy
- checking for extraintestinal complications
- colonoscopic cancer surveillance

Self-help (see Table 5.2)

Supportive treatment

Dietary and nutritional advice

Drugs

- antidiarrheal agents (not in active colitis)
- colestyramine (ileal disease or resection for Crohn's disease)
- hematinics (iron, folate, vitamin B_{12})
- vitamins, electrolytes
- osteoporosis prophylaxis and treatment
- heparin, administered subcutaneously (inpatients with active IBD)

Drugs to avoid

- antidiarrheal drugs (in active colitis)
- non-essential NSAIDs, antibiotics, delayed-release drugs

Specific treatment (according to presentation)

Drugs

- corticosteroids
- aminosalicylates
- immunomodulatory drugs (azathioprine/MP, ciclosporin, methotrexate)
- antibiotics
- cytokine therapy (infliximab, adalimumab, certolizumab pegol)
- other

Nutritional therapy (Crohn's disease only)

- liquid formula diet

Surgery

MP, mercaptopurine; NSAID, non-steroidal anti-inflammatory drug.

TABLE 5.2

Advice to help optimize self-management

Learn about IBD from:

- patient support groups
- books for patients about IBD
- websites and newspaper articles (but beware unreliable information sources)
- IBD specialist nurse
- hospital doctor

Look after yourself at home by:

- stopping smoking (especially if you have Crohn's disease)
- eating a balanced diet in general; following special dietary advice when recommended
- sticking rigorously to prescribed treatments; not stopping maintenance treatment because you are feeling well
- self-medicating for minor relapses using guidelines issued by hospital IBD team when available (especially ulcerative colitis)
- stopping a drug immediately and informing the hospital doctor or IBD nurse if a side effect is suspected
- avoiding drugs which may worsen IBD (e.g. NSAIDs, antibiotics) (unless essential)
- discussing complementary or alternative therapy with hospital IBD team if considering it, and not stopping conventional treatment
- joining patient support group and attending local meetings

Make the most of hospital care by:

- insisting on care by a specialist IBD team
- ensuring the hospital has an IBD nurse and not hesitating to telephone him/her when necessary
- not hesitating to ask hospital IBD team if uncertain about any aspect of illness, tests or treatment
- fixing *urgent* outpatient appointment if IBD is causing problems
- attending scheduled outpatient appointments
- having blood and other investigations done when/as necessary
- pressing for adequate local IBD service (e.g. through patient panel)

Hospital care. Patients with ulcerative colitis are best managed, whether as outpatients or during admission to hospital, by specialist gastroenterological medical, surgical, nursing and dietetic staff working in close collaboration, with access to stoma therapists and, if possible, a trained counselor. Specialist outpatient IBD clinics are the best way of providing patients with the necessary clinical expertise in the form of joint medical–surgical consultations with open access for prompt review in the event of relapse. Such clinics also offer:

- continuity of care
- appropriate clinical, endoscopic and laboratory monitoring of the disease and its treatment
- training for doctors and nurses
- a sufficient patient base for clinical trials.

Most primary care providers have fewer than five patients with IBD under their care; this limited experience of the disease means that they should not generally be expected to take primary responsibility for the long-term management of either ulcerative colitis or Crohn's disease. However, some patients with stable, inactive and limited disease can be followed safely by their family doctor. This arrangement is dependent on appropriate shared care guidelines as well as prompt open access to the hospital IBD clinic when necessary.

Dietary advice and nutritional support. Patients with ulcerative colitis do not usually need specific dietary advice, although a few (fewer than 5%) may find their condition improves if they avoid cows' milk, and some with proctitis and proximal constipation may benefit from fiber supplementation.

Specific nutritional deficiencies are less common in ulcerative colitis than in Crohn's disease, but should be corrected as necessary with appropriate supplements. Sick inpatients who are malnourished often need enteral and occasionally total parenteral nutrition. However, there is no evidence that enteral nutrition is itself an effective primary therapy in active ulcerative colitis, in contrast to small-bowel Crohn's disease.

Drugs. Iron and folic acid supplements are often needed, as are appropriate drugs for incipient or established osteoporosis (see

Chapter 2). Subcutaneous heparin is recommended for patients admitted with active ulcerative colitis to reduce the risk of arterial and venous thrombosis.

Drugs to avoid. Antidiarrheal (loperamide, codeine phosphate, diphenoxylate), opioid analgesic, antispasmodic and anticholinergic drugs should be avoided in active ulcerative colitis as they may provoke acute colonic dilation. NSAIDs, and occasionally antibiotics, may provoke relapse of ulcerative colitis (see Chapter 1), and should not be used unless essential.

Treatment of active ulcerative colitis

Treatment is determined by:
- the extent of disease
- the severity of the attack.

Knowledge of the extent of disease is particularly important in relation to the feasibility of effective topical therapy, while the severity of the attack defines not only the optimal type and route of therapy, but also whether the patient can be safely treated as an outpatient or needs urgent hospital admission.

Who needs hospital admission? Immediate admission is required for those with acute severe attacks of ulcerative colitis, defined primarily by clinical features (see Chapter 2). These include six or more bloody diarrheal stools daily, pyrexia and tachycardia (more than 90 beats/ minute). Such patients will usually be systemically unwell, may be anemic and may have lost weight; in very ill patients there may be abdominal tenderness and/or distension.

The decision to admit does not usually depend on the results of blood or other tests of disease severity, though these will often be abnormal (see 'Blood tests' on page 88).

It is also advisable to admit less sick patients who have not responded as outpatients to 2 weeks' treatment with oral prednisolone (see 'Active left-sided or extensive ulcerative colitis' on page 93). Since the initial attack of ulcerative colitis is more dangerous than subsequent ones, the threshold for admission should be lowered in those presenting for the first time with bloody diarrhea.

Inpatient management of acute severe ulcerative colitis

General measures. These patients should be admitted immediately to a gastroenterology ward for close joint medical, surgical and nursing care (Table 5.3). Early involvement of the nutrition team and of a stoma therapist in those likely to need surgery is important. All patients undergoing an acute attack of ulcerative colitis need to be kept fully informed of their treatment and its likely outcome; they need to be aware from the outset that they have a one in four chance of needing an urgent colectomy during their admission.

Establishing the diagnosis, extent of disease and its severity requires a carefully targeted history and appropriate investigations (see Chapter 3) in those presenting for the first time. In patients with established ulcerative colitis, these procedures are required to exclude infection and to assess disease extent (if not already known) and severity.

Clinical evaluation. In patients with established ulcerative colitis, direct questions about stool frequency, consistency and urgency, overt blood content, abdominal pain, malaise, fever and weight loss indicate the severity of the attack. External examination should include assessment of general health, pulse rate and temperature, as well as a check for anemia, fluid depletion, weight loss, and abdominal tenderness or distension.

The differential diagnosis may also need evaluation in those presenting with bloody diarrhea for the first time (see Table 3.1). Abrupt onset with fever, vomiting, epidemic or contact history and/or recent foreign travel suggests infective colitis, even in those with pre-existing ulcerative colitis. Cytomegalovirus (CMV) should be considered, particularly in patients known to be immunosuppressed. *C. difficile* infection is a mimic as well as common concomitant of attacks of ulcerative colitis, whether or not there has been previous antibiotic exposure, while NSAIDs may cause either a relapse of established IBD or de novo colitis (which usually remits rapidly on NSAID withdrawal). In patients presenting for the first time, non-smoking or recent cessation of smoking increases the likelihood of ulcerative colitis, while previous abdominal or pelvic irradiation make radiation colitis a strong possibility. Ischemic colitis usually shows sudden onset in older people with other features of

TABLE 5.3

Principles of inpatient management of acute severe ulcerative colitis

General measures

Explanation, psychosocial support

- physicians, specialist nurses
- patient support groups

Specialist multidisciplinary care

- physicians, surgeons, nutrition team, nurses, stoma therapist, counselor

Establishing the diagnosis, extent and severity

Clinical evaluation

Complete blood cell count, ESR, C-reactive protein, albumin, liver-function tests, amebic serology

Stool microscopy, culture, *Clostridium difficile* toxin

Sigmoidoscopy and biopsy

Plain abdominal X-ray

Consider colonoscopy, air or instant contrast enema, leukocyte scan

Monitoring progress

Daily clinical assessment

- abdominal examination (twice daily)
- stool chart
- 4-hourly temperature, pulse

Daily complete blood cell count, ESR, C-reactive protein, urea and electrolytes, albumin

Daily plain abdominal X-ray

Supportive treatment

Intravenous fluids, electrolytes, blood transfusion

Nutritional supplementation

Subcutaneous heparin

CONTINUED

TABLE 5.3 (CONTINUED)

Avoid antidiarrheals (codeine, loperamide, diphenoxylate), opiates, NSAIDs

Rolling maneuver (if colon dilating)

Specific treatments

Medical

- intravenous (hydrocortisone or methylprednisolone) then oral corticosteroids (prednisolone)
- continue with oral 5-ASA in patients already taking it; otherwise start when improvement begins
- antibiotics for very sick febrile patients, or when infection is suspected
- for patients not responding to steroids at 4–7 days, consider:
  - intravenous then oral ciclosporin (with trimethoprim–sulfamethoxazole prophylaxis) or
  - an infliximab infusion

Surgical (for non-responders at 5–7 days, toxic megacolon, perforation, massive hemorrhage)

- panproctocolectomy with ileoanal pouch or permanent ileostomy
- subtotal colectomy with ileorectal anastomosis (rarely)

5-ASA, 5-aminosalicylate; ESR, erythrocyte sedimentation rate; NSAIDs, non-steroidal anti-inflammatory drugs.

vascular disease, and often causes marked abdominal pain as well as bloody diarrhea. The very rare Behçet's enterocolitis may be suggested by a history of cyclic oral and genital ulceration, uveitis, erythema nodosum, pathergy (the formation of pustules at the site of minor trauma, such as venepuncture) and/or arthropathy.

Blood tests are better for establishing the activity of ulcerative colitis than for making the diagnosis or identifying its extent (see Chapter 3). The best laboratory measures of disease activity in ulcerative colitis are hemoglobin, platelet count, ESR, C-reactive protein and serum albumin. For recent travelers, serology as well as stool samples should be requested (for amebiasis, strongyloidiasis and schistosomiasis).

Sigmoidoscopy and rectal biopsy. Cautious rigid or flexible sigmoidoscopy and biopsy in the unprepared patient, and without excessive air insufflation, provides immediate confirmation of active colitis. Full colonoscopy may cause colonic perforation and dilation, and should be avoided in acute severe ulcerative colitis.

Plain abdominal X-ray at presentation is used to assess disease extent and activity, and to look for dilation. In patients with suspected colonic perforation, diagnosis can be confirmed by erect chest X-ray or a lateral decubitus abdominal film.

Radiolabeled leukocyte scans. ^{99}Tc-HMPAO scanning provides information about disease activity and particularly extent where doubt exists in patients with ulcerative colitis.

Monitoring progress. Progress is monitored by twice-daily clinical assessment, including:

- abdominal examination, particularly by percussion, for gaseous distension, loss of hepatic dullness (which may indicate free gas in the peritoneal cavity), and peritoneal irritation
- stool chart (recording frequency, consistency, presence of overt blood and urgency)
- 4-hourly measurement of temperature and pulse.

Blood count, ESR, C-reactive protein, routine biochemistry and plain abdominal X-ray should be undertaken daily in sick patients (Table 5.3).

Intravenous fluids and blood. Most patients require intravenous fluids and electrolytes, particularly potassium, to replace diarrheal losses. The serum potassium concentration should be maintained at or above 4 mmol/liter, since hypokalemia may predispose to colonic dilation. Blood transfusion is usually recommended if the hemoglobin level falls below 10 g/dL.

Nutritional support. Patients can usually eat normally, with liquid protein and calorie supplements if necessary. Very sick patients, many of whom will undergo surgery, may need enteral or parenteral nutrition.

Anticoagulation. Because active ulcerative colitis is associated with a high risk of venous and arterial thromboembolism, patients should be given prophylactic subcutaneous heparin (e.g. low-molecular-weight

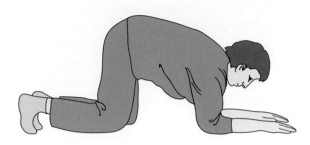

Figure 5.1 Knee–elbow position for rolling maneuver.

heparin, 3000–5000 units daily). Heparin does not appear to increase rectal blood loss, even when given intravenously.

Drugs to avoid are antidiarrheal (codeine phosphate, loperamide, diphenoxylate), opioid analgesic, antispasmodic and anticholinergic drugs, as well as NSAIDs. If mild pain relief is needed, oral paracetamol (acetaminophen) appears to be well tolerated, while severe pain suggests colonic dilation or perforation needing urgent evaluation and/or intervention.

Rolling maneuver. In very sick patients, particularly those with clinical and/or radiological evidence of incipient colonic dilation, rolling into the prone or knee–elbow position (Figure 5.1) for 15 minutes every 2 hours may aid in the evacuation of gas from the rectum, deflation of the colon and prevention of toxic megacolon.

Drug therapy. A possible management pathway is shown in Figure 5.2. Corticosteroids remain the cornerstone of specific medical treatment for acute severe ulcerative colitis. Aminosalicylates and antibiotics have minor roles. Ciclosporin or infliximab are useful in some steroid-refractory patients. However, oral azathioprine and mercaptopurine (MP) are too slow to work in those with acute steroid-refractory attacks.

Corticosteroids. Hydrocortisone (300–400 mg/day) or methylprednisolone (40–60 mg/day) are given intravenously. There is no advantage in giving higher doses, although continuous infusion may be more effective than once- or twice-daily boluses. Corticosteroid drip enemas (e.g. prednisolone, 20 mg, or hydrocortisone, 100 mg in

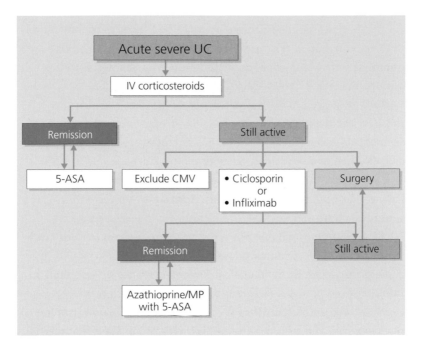

Figure 5.2 General principles of managing acute severe ulcerative colitis. In practice, each step will depend on detailed daily evaluation of the patient (see text) and discussion of the options under consideration. 5-ASA, 5-aminosalicylate; CMV, cytomegalovirus; IV, intravenous; MP, mercaptopurine; UC, ulcerative colitis.

100–200 mL water given rectally via a soft catheter twice daily with the patient in the left lateral position) are sometimes given in addition to intravenous steroids, but their value is unproven.

About 70% of patients who receive corticosteroids improve substantially in 5–7 days. They are then switched to oral prednisolone (40–60 mg/day), the dose being tapered to zero over 2–3 months. Formerly, failure to respond to intravenous steroids after 7 days indicated the need for urgent colectomy (see Chapter 7), but ciclosporin or infliximab are now alternatives.

Aminosalicylates at full dose, should be continued in those already taking them at the time of admission and who are well enough to take oral medication, but these drugs do not have a primary therapeutic effect in acute severe ulcerative colitis. In case patients given aminosalicylates for the first time prove to be allergic to or intolerant of them, initiation of this therapy is best delayed until the patient has improved sufficiently while receiving intravenous steroids to switch to oral treatment (see Tables 4.2 and 4.3).

Antibiotics are usually restricted to very sick febrile patients, or to those in whom an infective component is strongly suspected. Under such circumstances, a combination of antibiotics is often given (e.g. ciprofloxacin or a cephalosporin with metronidazole).

Ciclosporin. Intravenous ciclosporin, 2–4 mg/kg/day for 5 days, followed by oral ciclosporin (Neoral), 5 mg/kg/day, given with continued corticosteroids, averts colectomy in the acute phase in 60–80% of patients who do not respond to intravenous steroids given alone for 5–7 days. Oral trimethoprim–sulfamethoxazole may be coprescribed as prophylaxis against *Pneumocystis carinii* infection. Enthusiasm for this treatment has to be tempered both by the frequency of relapse necessitating colectomy (up to 50%) that follows withdrawal of ciclosporin, and by its serious adverse effects (see Table 4.5) which, in turn, demand frequent monitoring of ciclosporin blood levels and serum biochemistry.

Infliximab. Recent controlled data indicate that after a single infusion of infliximab, 5 mg/kg, the need for colectomy can be reduced from 70% to 30% in patients who have not improved with intravenous steroids alone. This response rate closely resembles that with ciclosporin (see above). Although it remains difficult to decide whether to recommend ciclosporin or infliximab for patients with steroid-refractory acute severe ulcerative colitis who are reluctant to have, or are unfit for, prompt surgery, the risk–benefit ratio probably lies in favor of infliximab.

Toxic megacolon. As mentioned earlier, the rolling maneuver may help to prevent toxic megacolon in very sick patients (see Figure 5.1). If the intensive treatment outlined in Table 5.3 (including rolling, intravenous antibiotics and a nasogastric tube to aspirate bowel gas and fluids) has not produced improvement in 24–48 hours – and if colonic dilation becomes established, particularly if associated with systemic toxicity – immediate surgery (see Chapter 7) is indicated.

Colonic perforation and massive hemorrhage are rare complications that require emergency surgery after appropriate urgent resuscitation, including intravenous antibiotics and blood transfusion, respectively (see Chapter 7). Even with immediate surgical intervention, the mortality of colonic perforation, which can occasionally also occur in patients without colonic dilation, is up to 30%.

Outcome. About 80% of patients with severe ulcerative colitis avoid colectomy in the acute phase when treated with intravenous corticosteroids (and ciclosporin or infliximab additionally if necessary). Of these, however, over 50% will have had a colectomy for recurrent episodes of active disease before 5 years has elapsed. Mortality of acute severe ulcerative colitis should now be under 3%.

Active left-sided or extensive ulcerative colitis (mild-to-moderate attack)

The principles of evaluation and management of mild-to-moderate attacks of ulcerative colitis (when the patient is well, with fewer than six stools daily) resemble those described above for inpatients (see Table 5.3); management is outlined in Figure 5.3. These patients, however, can usually be managed as outpatients. Stools should be sent to be checked for infection. In mild attacks of left-sided disease, an oral aminosalicylate (5-ASA) (see Table 4.2) with daily 5-ASA or steroid enemas may suffice. Often, however, oral prednisolone, 20–60 mg/day (the dose depending on the severity of the attack), is also needed for 2–3 weeks. The dose is then tapered by 5 mg every 5–10 days. Oral iron and/or folate may also be necessary.

Those who do not begin to respond to these measures within 2 weeks (10–40%) or who deteriorate often need prompt hospital admission for more intensive management, including intravenous steroids (see above and Table 5.3). An alternative approach in steroid-refractory patients who are not so acutely ill as to require hospital admission, and in whom a response to treatment taking up to 4 months is acceptable, is to introduce oral azathioprine, 2.0–2.5 mg/kg/day, or MP, 1.0–1.5 mg/kg/day, with appropriate laboratory monitoring (see Table 4.4). Patients who do not respond to, or who are intolerant of,

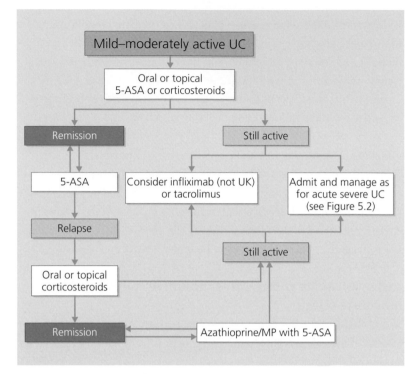

Figure 5.3 General principles of managing mild to moderately active ulcerative colitis. The route of administration of 5-ASA drugs and corticosteroids will depend on the extent of the colitis (see text). In practice, each step will depend on detailed evaluation of the patient (see text) and discussion of the options under consideration. 5-ASA, 5-aminosalicylate; MP, mercaptopurine; UC, ulcerative colitis.

thiopurines and who are unwilling to have a colectomy can be offered methotrexate (see page 66), while a further alternative, which is not permitted in all countries (see below), is to introduce regular infliximab infusions (see Table 4.6). Lastly, oral tacrolimus can be offered, though experience of this approach to date is limited (see page 70).

Active proctitis

The principles of the management of proctitis resemble those described for more extensive ulcerative colitis. Management aspects specific to distal disease are outlined here and in Table 5.4.

Establishing the diagnosis. The diagnosis of proctitis, together with its extent and severity, can usually be quickly confirmed by rigid or flexible sigmoidoscopy and biopsy. However, care needs to be taken not to mistake rectal Crohn's disease, cancer, polyps, benign solitary ulcer, hemorrhoids, anal fissure or 'gay bowel' for proctitis. In patients who prove difficult to treat, and depending on the clinical picture, other diagnoses such as irritable bowel syndrome (which may coexist with proctitis), celiac disease, collagenous colitis, NSAID-induced colitis and 5-ASA intolerance should also be considered.

Supportive treatment. Rarely, patients benefit from avoiding cows' milk or other food components that they have noticed provoke attacks. In

TABLE 5.4

Principles of the treatment of active proctitis

Supportive treatment

Treat proximal constipation with fiber and/or a laxative (e.g. magnesium hydroxide)

Avoid cows' milk or other specific food (rarely)

Specific treatment

Topical 5-ASA or, as second line, steroids (suppository, liquid or foam enema)

Oral 5-ASA

Refractory proctitis

Oral or intravenous steroids

Oral azathioprine or MP

Acetarsol suppositories

Other possibilities: ciclosporin, lidocaine or short-chain fatty acid enemas, nicotine patches or enemas

Surgery: total proctocolectomy

5-ASA, 5-aminosalicylate; MP, mercaptopurine.

those with proximal constipation, a high-fiber diet, oral fiber supplements and/or a stool-softening laxative such as macrogol may be helpful. It is conceivable that alleviation of constipation may improve the symptoms of proctitis, at least in part, by increasing the delivery of orally administered 5-ASA to the rectum.

Specific medical treatment. Depending on disease extent, suppositories or enemas of 5-ASA (see Table 4.3) or corticosteroids (see Table 4.1) are inserted once or twice daily until about 2 weeks after bleeding subsides. Suppositories reach about 100 mm from the anal margin, foam enemas 200 mm and liquid enemas, with optimal patient positioning, the splenic flexure. Topical treatment with 5-ASA preparations is more effective than with corticosteroids. Although prednisolone metasulfobenzoate and budesonide enemas suppress adrenal function to a lesser extent than other topical steroids, the choice of product for routine use depends on patient preference in relation to ease of insertion and retention, foam often being favored on both counts.

In patients with recurrent attacks, an oral aminosalicylate (see Table 4.2) is added, in part to initiate subsequent remission maintenance in those who prefer long-term oral to rectal treatment. Balsalazide and olsalazine, which deliver 5-ASA exclusively to the colon, may be preferable to slow-release or pH-dependent delayed-release aminosalicylates, which release 5-ASA more proximally.

Refractory proctitis

Up to 80% of patients respond in 2–4 weeks to the measures described for treating active proctitis. In those who do not respond, the diagnosis needs careful confirmation. Alternative approaches in refractory proctitis, which can sometimes be very difficult to treat, include full-dose oral or even intravenous corticosteroids, and oral azathioprine, 2.0–2.5 mg/kg/day, or MP, 1.0–1.5 mg/kg/day. Suppositories containing arsenic (acetarsol) may induce remission in distal disease but, because of the risk of systemic arsenic toxicity, should only be used for short-term management (up to 4 weeks). More experimental options include ciclosporin, short-chain fatty acid or lidocaine enemas, and nicotine patches or enemas (see Table 4.7). None of the enemas listed is commercially available yet, but many hospital pharmacies will prepare them if requested.

Many patients will feel angry about their disease and their doctor's failure to rectify their symptoms; some may need counseling. In exceptional cases, all medical treatments fail, and patients require panproctocolectomy (see Chapter 7). Left-sided colonic resections in ulcerative colitis are too frequently followed by recurrence in the residual colon to be a practical option.

Maintaining remission

5-ASAs. Patients with disease of limited extent and relapses occurring less than once a year may decline maintenance therapy. However, most require an oral aminosalicylate for life (Table 4.2) with appropriate blood checks every 6–12 months (Table 4.3). Such therapy reduces the annual relapse rate to 20–30% from 70–80% with no treatment. To minimize possible systemic side effects, some patients with recurrent attacks of distal disease may prefer topical prophylactic 5-ASA therapy, with enemas or suppositories once or twice daily or even three times weekly.

Azathioprine and MP. In those who relapse repeatedly despite a 5-ASA in adequate dosage, and/or whenever steroid therapy after acute episodes is withdrawn, oral azathioprine, 2.0–2.5 mg/kg/day, or MP, 1.0–1.5 mg/kg/day, carefully monitored (Table 4.4) and given for at least 2 years, is of proven benefit. How long the therapy should be maintained for patients with ulcerative colitis is unclear. It may be prudent to attempt to discontinue it after 4–5 years without relapse.

Infliximab. Two recent trials suggest that infusions of infliximab, 5 mg/kg every 8 weeks, may be useful in maintaining remission in some patients with ulcerative colitis that is poorly controlled by steroids and/or thiopurines. Whether the benefit obtained with infliximab in this context outweighs its side effects and justifies its cost (see Chapter 4) is not yet clear: indeed in the UK, for example, the National Institute for Health and Clinical Excellence does not advocate use of infliximab in this setting.

Surgery. Occasionally, patients continue to have active ulcerative colitis despite all the measures described above. These, particularly if steroid-dependent, require proctocolectomy (Chapter 7).

Follow-up

Patients with well-controlled distal ulcerative colitis can be followed routinely by the primary care provider, subject to referral for colonoscopy at 8–10 years to reassess disease extent in relation to the possible need for cancer surveillance (see below). They should also be referred promptly to a gastroenterologist if they do not respond to treatment for relapse.

All other patients require periodic review (every 6–12 months if in remission) in a specialized hospital clinic offering immediate open access in the event of relapse. Such arrangements ensure continuity of care and optimal monitoring of the disease, its complications and its treatment. At routine outpatient appointments, disease activity is assessed by questions about bowel habit, quality of life and time off work; sigmoidoscopy is reserved for those in whom the history suggests active disease.

Surveillance for colorectal cancer. The increased risk of colorectal cancer in chronic extensive ulcerative colitis (see Chapter 2) has led to the introduction of colonoscopic surveillance programs. Conventionally, at least 30 biopsies from randomly selected sites throughout the colon, and from any raised lesions, have been recommended every 1–3 years, depending on the duration of the disease, and starting 8–10 years after onset.

Many clinicians, however, believe that careful inspection is more important than the total number of blind biopsies taken. The earlier conservative recommendation is time-consuming and tedious not only for the patient and colonoscopist, but particularly for the pathologist examining the multiple biopsies. New colonoscopic techniques undergoing evaluation include high-definition and magnifying colonoscopy, and use of dye-spray (Figure 5.4), narrow-band imaging and autofluorescence during the procedure. All these methods provide improved identification and definition of tiny mucosal abnormalities, so

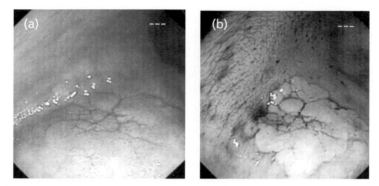

Figure 5.4 Colonoscopic views of mucosal dysplastic lesion seen:
(a) before; and (b) after spraying the mucosa with indigo carmine.
Reproduced courtesy of Dr M Rutter, University Hospital of North Tees,
Stockton-on-Tees, UK.

that biopsies can be targeted directly at lesions previously easily missed:
such techniques give a much higher 'hit rate' for dysplasia, obviate the
need for multiple random biopsies and thereby substantially reduce the
pathologist's workload.

Lastly, a few centers are assessing confocal endomicroscopy, in which
microscopic images of suspicious areas of gut mucosa are obtained
during the colonoscopy, thereby potentially diagnosing dysplasia or
cancer during the test itself.

If biopsies show the premalignant changes of high-grade epithelial
dysplasia (Figure 5.5), colectomy is indicated (Chapter 7). In those with
confirmed low-grade dysplasia, colectomy or, for those reluctant to
have surgery, more frequent colonoscopic surveillance is recommended,
because the incidence of cancer in this situation is about 50% in 5 years.
Unfortunately, surveillance programs have not been shown to reduce
mortality from colonic cancer in ulcerative colitis, in part because
about 25% of cancers occur in patients without detected, preceding
or associated dysplasia.

Molecular biological techniques (e.g. looking for DNA aneuploidy,
p53 heterozygosity) are likely, in due course, to supersede dependence
on the colonoscopic detection of dysplasia for the prevention of
colorectal cancer in ulcerative colitis.

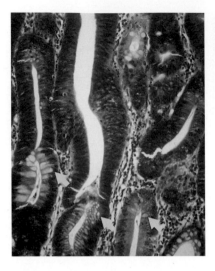

Figure 5.5 Severe epithelial dysplasia in ulcerative colitis, showing glandular distortion, stratification of the epithelium with heaping of nuclei, and nuclear polymorphism and hyperchromaticism. Note the normal crypts at the bottom of the picture (arrowed).
Photomicrograph courtesy of Professor RM Feakins, Barts and The London School of Medicine and Dentistry, London, UK.

Colitis of uncertain type or etiology

Acute CUTE, in which the clinical, endoscopic and histological features of the disease do not allow its definite classification as either ulcerative colitis or Crohn's colitis (see Chapter 2), is managed like acute severe ulcerative colitis. However, in patients coming to surgery, it is usually advisable to avoid the immediate formation of an ileoanal pouch, in view of the high risk of pouch failure if the diagnosis proves to be Crohn's disease (see Chapter 7).

Key points – medical management of ulcerative colitis

- The treatment of ulcerative colitis depends on disease extent and severity.
- Active ulcerative colitis is treated primarily with corticosteroids and aminosalicylates, with ciclosporin, infliximab or surgery for refractory acute severe disease.
- Maintenance of remission in ulcerative colitis is usually achieved with aminosalicylates, although thiopurines are required for those in whom aminosalicylates are ineffective.
- Patients with ulcerative colitis should participate in decisions about their treatment, particularly in relation to possible surgery.

Key references

Azad-Khan AK, Piris J, Truelove SC. An experiment to determine the active moiety of sulphasalazine. *Lancet* 1977;2:892–5.

Carter MJ, Lobo AJ, Travis SP. IBD Section, British Society of Gastroenterology. Guidelines for the management of inflammatory bowel disease in adults. *Gut* 2004;53 (suppl 5):V1–16.

Hawthorne AB, Logan RF, Hawkey CJ et al. Randomised controlled trial of azathioprine withdrawal in ulcerative colitis. *BMJ* 1992;305: 20–2.

Järnerot G, Hertervig E, Friis-Liby I et al. Infliximab as rescue therapy in severe to moderately severe ulcerative colitis: a randomised, placebo-controlled study. *Gastroenterology* 2005;128:1805–11.

Kiesslich R, Galle PR, Neurath MF. Endoscopic surveillance in ulcerative colitis: smart biopsies do it better. *Gastroenterology* 2007;133:742–5.

Kornbluth A, Sachar DB. Ulcerative colitis practice guidelines in adults (update). American College of Gastroenterology, Practice Parameters Committee. *Am J Gastroenterol* 2004;99:1371–85.

Lichtiger S, Present DH, Kornbluth A et al. Cyclosporine in severe ulcerative colitis refractory to steroid therapy. *N Engl J Med* 1994;330:1841–5.

Rutgeerts P, Sandborn WJ, Feagan BG et al. Infliximab for induction and maintenance therapy for ulcerative colitis. *N Engl J Med* 2005;353:2462–76.

Sutherland L, Roth D, Beck P, Makiyama K. Oral 5-aminosalicylic acid for maintenance of remission in ulcerative colitis. *Cochrane Database Syst Rev* 2002;4:CD000544. www.thecochranelibrary.com

Travis SPL, Stange EF, Lémann M et al for the European Crohn's and Colitis Organisation (ECCO). European Consensus on the diagnosis and management of ulcerative colitis: current management. *J Crohn's and Colitis* 2008;2:24–62.

Truelove SC, Witts LJ. Cortisone in ulcerative colitis. Final report on a therapeutic trial. *BMJ* 1955;2: 1041–8.

Treatment of Crohn's disease not only depends on disease activity and site, as in ulcerative colitis, but also needs to be tailored according to the individual's clinical presentation and dominant underlying pathological explanation. Inflammation, obstruction, abscess and fistula require different therapeutic approaches, and they often need to be distinguished by appropriate investigation before specific treatment is begun. Drug therapy in Crohn's disease is generally less effective than in ulcerative colitis, and dietary and surgical treatment correspondingly more important.

General measures

Explanation, psychosocial support and hospital care. Newly diagnosed patients with Crohn's disease, as with ulcerative colitis, need a full explanation of their illness, preferably assisted by the written information provided by patient support groups (see Chapter 5, Table 5.1 and the 'Useful resources' section). A substantial minority of patients are sufficiently disturbed psychologically by the chronically disabling nature of their illness to need more formal psychosocial help. As with ulcerative colitis, out- and in-patient care is best undertaken by a specialist multidisciplinary hospital team.

Dietary advice and nutritional support. All patients should be carefully assessed in relation to their nutritional intake and status, the latter clinically by measurement of weight, height and then body mass index (BMI = weight [kg]/height [m]^2; normal BMI > 20).

Patients with stricturing small-bowel Crohn's disease should avoid high-residue foods (e.g. citrus fruit, nuts, sweetcorn, uncooked vegetables) that might cause bolus obstruction. Special dietary and nutritional modifications are needed for those with extensive small-bowel Crohn's disease, or short-bowel syndrome (see Chapter 2). Sick inpatients may need enteral or parenteral nutrition to restore nutritional deficits, while liquid formula diets provide a primary therapy option for some with active small-bowel Crohn's disease.

Non-specific drugs. Diarrhea in Crohn's disease has a number of different causes, each requiring a different therapeutic approach (see Table 2.1). Codeine phosphate and loperamide are often useful for the symptomatic control of diarrhea that is due to active disease or previous bowel resection. As in active ulcerative colitis, however, they should be avoided in active Crohn's colitis in case they provoke colonic dilation.

Colestyramine, 4 g one to three times daily, is often helpful in patients with Crohn's disease complicated by bile-salt-induced diarrhea as a result of extensive terminal ileal disease or resection (see 'Bile-salt malabsorption' on page 131). By binding bile salts, colestyramine may, however, exacerbate or induce steatorrhea and malabsorption of fat-soluble vitamins; it may also directly bind with and prevent the absorption of other drugs and should not, therefore, be given simultaneously with other therapies.

Hematinics (iron, folate and vitamin B_{12}), calcium, magnesium, zinc and fat-soluble vitamins (A, D, E and K) may be needed for the replacement of particular deficiencies, as may appropriate drugs for incipient or established osteoporosis (see Chapter 2). In patients with iron-deficiency anemia who are intolerant of, or not responsive to, oral iron supplements, intravenous iron preparations such as ferric carboxymaltose, iron sucrose and low molecular weight iron dextran are safe and usually effective. Subcutaneous heparin to reduce the risk of arterial and venous thrombosis is recommended for those admitted with active Crohn's disease.

Drugs to avoid. NSAIDs may precipitate relapse of Crohn's disease and should, if possible, be avoided. Likewise, in patients with small-bowel stricturing due to Crohn's disease, delayed-release drugs should not be prescribed in case they cause bolus obstruction. Anecdotal evidence suggests that iron salts can exacerbate relapses, and their prescription is best postponed until remission has been achieved. In those who are frequently hospitalized because of pain, use of opioids should be minimized to avoid narcotic addiction.

Treatment of active Crohn's disease

Who needs hospital admission? The heterogeneous presentation of
Crohn's disease makes assessment of disease activity more complicated
than in ulcerative colitis. For clinical trials, a large number of
multifactorial clinical and/or laboratory-based scoring systems, such
as the Crohn's Disease Activity Index (CDAI), has been devised, but
none is suitable for ordinary clinical use. The working definitions of the
American College of Gastroenterology (Table 6.1) are more practical.
Many patients with active Crohn's disease can be looked after as
outpatients, but those with moderate-to-severe and severe-to-fulminant
disease need prompt, and in the latter instance immediate, hospital
admission. In patients with Crohn's colitis, indications for admission
resemble those for acute severe ulcerative colitis (see Chapter 5).

TABLE 6.1

**American College of Gastroenterology's working definition of
disease activity in Crohn's disease**

Activity	Features
Remission	Asymptomatic patients
Mild to moderate	Outpatients able to take oral nutrition, with symptoms but no fluid depletion, fever, abdominal tenderness, painful mass or obstruction
Moderate to severe	Patients who have not responded to treatment of mild to moderate disease, or those with more prominent symptoms including fever, weight loss > 10%, abdominal pain or tenderness (without rebound), intermittent nausea or vomiting (without obstructive findings) or anemia
Severe to fulminant	Patients with persisting symptoms despite outpatient oral steroids, or those with high fever, persistent vomiting, intestinal obstruction, rebound tenderness, cachexia or abscess

Adapted from Hanauer SB, Meyers S. *Am J Gastroenterol* 2001;96:635–43.

General measures. As for those with ulcerative colitis, patients with active Crohn's disease should be looked after by a multidisciplinary team with special expertise in IBD in a specialist gastroenterology clinic or ward (see Table 5.1). Options for treatment (medical, nutritional, surgical) are wider than in ulcerative colitis, and it is essential that the patient with Crohn's disease is kept fully informed about his or her illness, and takes a place at the center of the therapeutic decision-making process.

Establishing the diagnosis, clinicopathological problem and severity. For many patients, the diagnosis of Crohn's disease and identification of its principal site will have been made before he or she presents with a relapse. Investigations, therefore, are directed primarily at clarifying the dominant clinicopathological process so as to optimize subsequent treatment. In individuals presenting acutely for the first time, the diagnosis must be established (Table 6.2; see also Tables 3.1–3.4).

Clinical evaluation. Symptoms of active terminal ileal and ileocecal Crohn's disease are described in Chapter 2. Where the diagnosis of Crohn's disease has not yet been made, acute appendicitis with a mass may be particularly hard to differentiate from Crohn's disease, except with laparoscopy or laparotomy. In elderly patients presenting de novo, cecal carcinoma and lymphoma need careful consideration, while in some ethnic groups, for example South Asians, ileocecal tuberculosis must be excluded.

In Crohn's colitis, diarrhea is a more prominent symptom than pain; questions to be asked of previously undiagnosed patients are outlined in the section on acute severe ulcerative colitis in Chapter 5. External abdominal or perianal fistulas are usually clinically obvious, but direct questions may be necessary to identify enterovesical or enterovaginal fistulas.

Blood tests. As in ulcerative colitis, the main value of blood tests is in assessing and monitoring disease activity, which is related directly to the platelet count, ESR and C-reactive protein, and inversely to serum albumin. However, in very sick patients, particularly those with extensive small-bowel disease and steatorrhea, there may be laboratory evidence of malnutrition and malabsorption (anemia and low levels of

TABLE 6.2

Management of active ileocecal Crohn's disease

General measures

Explanation, psychosocial support

- physicians, specialist nurses
- patient support groups

Specialist multidisciplinary care

- physicians, surgeons, nutritionists, nurses, counselor

Establishing the diagnosis, site, extent and severity

Clinical evaluation

- complete blood cell count, ESR, C-reactive protein, ferritin, folate, B_{12}, albumin, liver-function tests, calcium, magnesium, zinc
- stool microscopy, culture, *Clostridium difficile* toxin
- plain abdominal X-ray
- consider ileocolonoscopy and biopsy, small-bowel barium radiology, ultrasound, CT scan, MRI, leukocyte scan

Monitoring progress

Daily clinical assessment

Stool chart

4-hourly temperature, pulse

Alternate daily complete blood cell count, ESR, C-reactive protein, urea and electrolytes, albumin

Daily plain abdominal X-ray (in patients with obstruction)

Supportive treatment

Fluids, electrolytes (sodium, potassium), blood transfusion

Nutritional supplementation; low-residue diet if small-bowel strictures

Subcutaneous heparin

Hematinics (B_{12}, folate)

Analgesia, antidiarrheals

Avoid NSAIDs, delayed-release drugs

(CONTINUED)

TABLE 6.2 (CONTINUED)

Specific treatments (separately or in combination)

Medical

- intravenous (hydrocortisone or methylprednisolone) then oral corticosteroids (prednisolone or budesonide)
- continue high-dose mesalazine in patients already taking it; otherwise consider starting when improvement begins
- consider metronidazole, ciprofloxacin, clarithromycin
- consider azathioprine/MP (slow responders) or infliximab for steroid non-responders

Nutritional

- liquid formula diet

Surgical

- resection or stricturoplasty

CT, computed tomography; ESR, erythrocyte sedimentation rate; MP, mercaptopurine; MRI, magnetic resonance imaging; NSAID, non-steroidal anti-inflammatory drug.

serum iron, folate, B_{12}, albumin, calcium, magnesium, zinc and essential fatty acids). A raised neutrophil count suggests intra-abdominal abscess, but corticosteroids also cause leukocytosis by demarginating intravascular neutrophils.

Stool microbiology. As in ulcerative colitis (see page 86), diarrhea in Crohn's disease may be due to intercurrent infection, particularly with C. *difficile* toxin. Stool samples should therefore be sent for microbiological analysis in all patients presenting with a recent onset of diarrhea.

Endoscopy and biopsy. In those with right iliac fossa pain where the diagnosis of Crohn's disease is in doubt, colonoscopy to the terminal ileum, with appropriate biopsies, can be helpful. It can also be used to balloon-dilate short strictures. In established Crohn's colitis, colonoscopy during acute relapse is not routinely necessary and may be unsafe, as in active ulcerative colitis (Chapter 5). In previously undiagnosed patients, digital rectal examination and cautious sigmoidoscopy may show rectal induration or ulceration, or the presence of perianal disease. Furthermore, biopsies of macroscopically normal rectal mucosa may reveal epithelioid granulomas in a minority of patients with more proximal Crohn's disease.

Plain abdominal X-ray. A plain film is essential if intestinal obstruction is suspected. It may also show a mass in the right iliac fossa and, in active Crohn's colitis, provide information about disease extent and severity.

Barium radiology. Because it may exacerbate obstructive symptoms and pre-existing perforation, conventional barium follow through and small-bowel enema should be avoided in severely ill patients with small-bowel disease; CT scanning or MRI are better alternatives. Contrast fistulography is useful in those with abdominal sinuses or fistulas.

Radiolabeled leukocyte scans. ^{99}Tc-HMPAO scanning can help to identify, non-invasively, not only sites of intestinal inflammation, as in ulcerative colitis, but also intra-abdominal abscesses in those with fever and/or an abdominal mass (see Chapter 3).

Ultrasound, CT scan and MRI. Abdominal ultrasound and a CT scan can be very useful in active Crohn's disease for the evaluation and percutaneous drainage of localized collections (see Chapter 3). Endoluminal ultrasound and MRI (Figure 6.1) are useful for the anatomic delineation of perianal abscesses and fistulas.

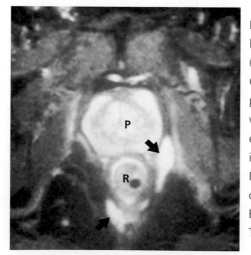

Figure 6.1 MRI showing a high-intensity signal track (arrowed) in a patient with Crohn's disease, indicating a posterior perianal collection with a fistulous track extending into the left ischiorectal fossa. P, prostate; R, rectum. Reproduced courtesy of Dr A McLean, Barts and The London NHS Trust, London, UK.

Supportive treatment. Patients with active Crohn's disease, like those with acute severe ulcerative colitis, need meticulous supportive treatment, including as necessary:

- intravenous fluids and electrolytes
- blood transfusion
- prophylactic subcutaneous heparin.

General nutritional and dietary measures, drug therapy and drugs to avoid are outlined in Table 6.2.

Active ileocecal Crohn's disease

Therapeutic options include drugs, a liquid formula diet and surgery (see Chapter 7), as separate alternatives or in combination, depending on the patient's age, presentation and personal preference (see Table 6.2). The possible treatment pathway is shown in Figure 6.2.

Drug therapy. *Corticosteroids.* In active disease, 60–80% of patients show symptomatic improvement when given oral steroids. Conventionally, prednisolone, 40–60 mg/day, is used, the dose being tapered by 5 mg every 7–10 days once improvement has begun, usually after 3–4 weeks. Very sick patients or those needing to fast because of intestinal obstruction need intravenous corticosteroids at least initially (e.g. hydrocortisone, 300–400 mg/day; methylprednisolone, 40–60 mg/day). In those able to take oral treatment in whom systemic steroid side effects are a major problem, budesonide (controlled ileal release, 9 mg/day) can be used, albeit at greater financial cost. It is important, however, to avoid giving any form of corticosteroid to patients with fistulating disease or an existing abscess because of the risk of producing or exacerbating sepsis (see Chapter 4).

Up to 20% of patients with Crohn's disease may be difficult to wean off steroids after relapse. Of these, many will be able partially or totally to discontinue steroid therapy on the introduction of an immunomodulatory agent, or after surgical resection of short-segment disease. Those unable to discontinue steroids altogether and who are unsuitable for surgery should be offered anti-TNF therapy; only a tiny minority cannot be weaned off steroids altogether thereafter.

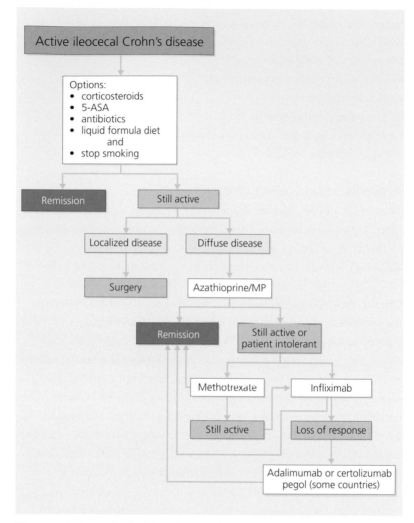

Figure 6.2 General principles of managing active Crohn's disease. In practice, each step will depend on detailed daily evaluation of the individual (see text) and discussion of the options under consideration. 5-ASA, 5-aminosalicylate; MP, mercaptopurine.

Aminosalicylates. Patients with only moderately active ileocecal disease, most of whom can be managed as outpatients, can be tried on high-dose oral mesalazine; about 40% will go into remission in 2–3 months.

Metronidazole and ciprofloxacin are modestly effective in mild to moderately active colonic Crohn's disease, but they are insufficiently potent for use as sole therapy in patients who are ill enough to need admission. Reports of the efficacy of clarithromycin and rifabutin, alone or in combination, need confirmation.

Immunosuppressive drugs. Patients who do not respond to corticosteroids, or relapse on their withdrawal, and who need to avoid operative treatment if possible because of extensive disease or previous surgery, can be treated with adjunctive oral azathioprine, 2.0–2.5 mg/kg/day, or MP, 1.0–1.5 mg/kg/day, the dose of steroids being reduced and/or phased out altogether as remission is achieved. Such patients must be well enough to wait for up to 4 months for this to occur. The side effects of azathioprine and MP make frequent blood counts and liver-function tests mandatory (see Chapter 4 and Table 4.4).

Azathioprine and MP are long-term options for Crohn's disease. However, in patients maintained in full remission on azathioprine or 6-MP, the risk of relapse after 4 years of treatment appears to be similar whether the drug is continued or stopped. In view of the potential toxicity associated with long-term use of these drugs, their withdrawal should be considered for those who are still in remission after 4 years of treatment.

Methotrexate is effective in about 40% of patients with steroid-refractory Crohn's disease when given intramuscularly or orally once a week. Its use is usually reserved for those who are unresponsive to, or intolerant of, thiopurines, and it requires appropriate monitoring (see Chapter 4).

Infliximab, 5 mg/kg, is used for patients with Crohn's disease refractory to steroids and/or conventional immunomodulatory drugs, and for whom surgery is inappropriate (see Chapter 4, Table 4.6). In this group, a three-dose induction regimen over 6 weeks produces remission (CDAI < 150) in about one-third of patients, and a substantial improvement in another third. Most patients are maintained on regular 8-weekly infusions thereafter, in conjunction with an immunomodulatory drug such as azathioprine for the first 6 months (see page 72). In patients who become asymptomatic on infliximab it is advisable to reassess their disease activity – for example with ileocolonoscopy – after about a year. Consideration can be given to stopping infliximab for those who are in complete remission endoscopically, with a beneficial effect on the risk of side effects, as well as on health costs.

Many patients lose their response to infliximab after a few weeks or months. In some, the effect is restored by a single infusion of 10 mg/kg or by a reduction in the interval between infusions. If these measures are ineffective, it is important to re-investigate to define the cause of symptoms. If they prove to be due to persisting disease too extensive to be operable, a switch to adalimumab, given every 2 weeks, can be helpful. For those losing response to adalimumab, the injections can be increased to weekly. In some countries, such as the USA, a third anti-TNFα antibody, certolizumab pegol, can be tried (page 71).

Dietary therapy. In patients with a poor response to corticosteroids, or a preference for avoiding them, in those with extensive small-bowel disease, and in children (see Chapter 8), a liquid formula diet is an alternative primary therapy. This can be either elemental (amino-acid based), oligomeric protein hydrolysate (containing peptides) or polymeric protein (containing whole protein and not, therefore, hypoallergenic), and is usually given for 4–6 weeks as the sole nutritional source (Table 6.3).

This approach is probably as effective as corticosteroid therapy in the short term, as about 60% of patients achieve remission. Unfortunately, after the resumption of a normal diet, many patients relapse (50% at 6 months). Whether this can be prevented by the selective and gradual reintroduction of particular low-fat, low-fiber foods to which individual patients are not intolerant, or by the intermittent use of further enteral feeding for short periods, remains to be proven.

The success of enteral nutrition as a primary therapy for Crohn's disease is also limited by:
- its cost
- the unpleasant taste of some of the available preparations
- the frequent need to give the feed by nasogastric tube
- poor concordance with the necessary feeding regimen.

TABLE 6.3

Enteral nutrition in Crohn's disease

Indications

Active small-bowel Crohn's disease

Undernutrition in IBD

Preparations

Elemental, oligomeric, polymeric

Side effects

Intolerance	Taste, boredom, nasogastric tube, nausea
Diarrhea	Concurrent antibiotics, hyperosmolality, too fast administration
Metabolic	Fluid overload or depletion, hypo- or hyperglycemia, low sodium/potassium/phosphate

Pulmonary aspiration

Placement difficulties

Monitoring

Fluid balance chart

Twice-weekly weight, urea and electrolytes, glucose, albumin

Contraindications

Severe diarrhea

Patient refusal

Mechanisms of action (all speculative)

Hypoallergenic

Bowel rest

Altered bacterial flora

Reduced gut permeability

Altered gut immunity

Nutritional repletion (including essential micronutrients)

Nevertheless, such therapy does offer a valuable alternative in the well-motivated minority of adults for whom it is appropriate.

Surgery (limited right hemicolectomy) is indicated in the 20–40% of patients whose ileocecal disease does not respond to drug or dietary therapy, particularly if they have short-segment (less than 200 mm) rather than extensive disease (see Chapter 7). Indeed, some patients prefer surgery to the prospect of pharmacological or nutritional treatment of uncertain duration. There are no controlled data to confirm which approach is best. After surgery, there is a 50% chance of recurrent symptoms at 5 years and of further surgery at 10 years; taking a long-term aminosalicylate and/or thiopurine and stopping smoking may reduce these risks by up to 50%.

Specific treatment of other presentations of active Crohn's disease

The general principles of the management of other presentations of active Crohn's disease are the same as those described above. Specific aspects of management are outlined below.

Obstructive small-bowel Crohn's disease. In patients presenting with obstructive symptoms and signs (Chapter 2), and with corresponding abnormalities on plain abdominal X-ray (Figure 6.3), the principal difficulty lies in deciding whether stricturing is due to active inflammation, fibrosis with scarring or even adhesions. Sometimes laboratory markers (e.g. raised platelet count, ESR, C-reactive protein) and/or radiolabeled leukocyte scans can help to identify individuals with active inflammatory Crohn's disease, but in most instances a short trial of intravenous corticosteroids is given in addition to intravenous fluids and, if necessary, nasogastric suction (Table 6.4). Parenteral nutrition is required if resumption of an oral diet is not likely in 5–7 days.

If the stricture is in the upper jejunum, terminal ileum or colon, enteroscopic or colonoscopic balloon dilation can be undertaken (Figure 6.4). In patients who do not settle after 48–72 hours of conservative treatment, surgery is needed; the options are local

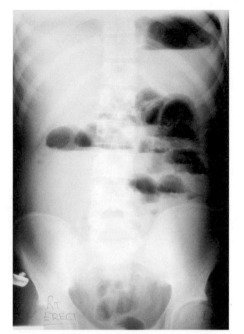

Figure 6.3 Plain abdominal X-ray showing small-bowel obstruction due to terminal ileal stricturing in Crohn's disease.

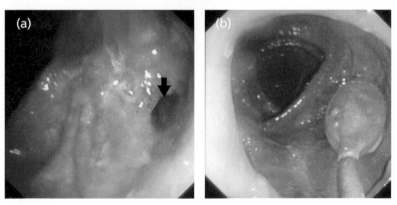

Figure 6.4 Colonoscopic balloon dilation of an anastomotic stricture in Crohn's disease: (a) narrowed ileocolonic anastomosis (arrowed); (b) through-the-scope balloon inserted into stricture and inflated.

resection or, for short and/or multiple strictures, stricturoplasty (see Chapter 7). Those responding to conservative therapy should be advised to take a low-residue diet to reduce the chance of recurrent symptoms.

TABLE 6.4

Specific treatments for other presentations of active Crohn's disease*

Subacute obstruction	Trial of intravenous corticosteroids
	Intravenous fluids and nasogastric suction (if necessary)
	Surgery for non-responders: local resection or stricturoplasty
Intra-abdominal abscess	Broad-spectrum antibiotics
	Percutaneous or surgical drainage
Intestinal fistula	Enteral or parenteral nutrition
	Oral metronidazole (for up to 3 months)
	Oral azathioprine or MP
	Consider infliximab infusions
	Surgery: local resection
Perianal disease	Oral metronidazole (for up to 3 months), ciprofloxacin
	Oral azathioprine or MP
	Infliximab infusions
	Surgery: drain abscesses, seton sutures for chronic fistulas
Oral and upper GI disease	Treat as in other sites
	Oral, topical or intralesional corticosteroids
	Omeprazole for duodenal disease

*Presentations other than ileocecal disease (Table 6.2) or Crohn's colitis (Table 6.5). GI, gastrointestinal; MP, mercaptopurine.

Intra-abdominal abscess. Ultrasound, CT, MRI and/or radiolabeled leukocyte scans are usually used to confirm the diagnosis of intra-abdominal abscess in patients with Crohn's disease who present with pain, weight loss, diarrhea and fever with or without a tender mass (Figure 6.5). Broad-spectrum antibiotics are given and the abscess drained either percutaneously under radiological control, and/or

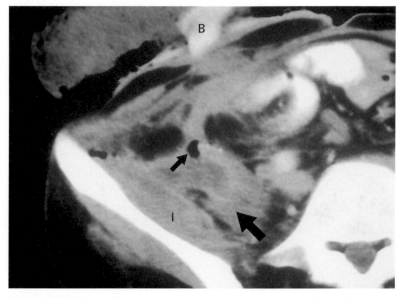

Figure 6.5 CT scan showing a psoas abscess in a patient with an ileostomy after total colectomy for Crohn's disease. Note the ileostomy bag (B) on the anterior abdominal wall with a short fistula (small arrow) leading from dilated prestomal small bowel into an abscess in psoas muscle (large arrow) adjacent to iliacus (I). Reproduced courtesy of Dr A McLean, Barts and The London NHS Trust, London, UK.

surgically (Table 6.4). When oral food intake is likely to be restricted for more than 5 days, parenteral nutrition should be started. Subsequent treatment is usually of the underlying pathological process, for example ileocecal inflammation.

Intestinal fistula. The relevant anatomic connections are clarified using contrast radiology, CT scans, endoluminal ultrasound and/or MRI (see 'Establishing the diagnosis' on page 105). Nutritional well-being should be restored using enteral or parenteral nutrition (Table 6.4). Where there is no obstruction distal to the site of intestinal fistulas, medical therapy with oral, rectal or intravenous metronidazole and/or oral azathioprine or MP will cause some fistulas to heal. Infliximab is a newer option, but its efficacy in closing fistulas that are not perianal is limited. Almost all patients with enterourinary or enterovaginal fistulas, 117 and most with enterocutaneous fistulas, require surgical resection of the fistula and local resection of involved intestine and/or other viscera (see Chapter 7).

Perianal disease. Non-suppurative perianal Crohn's disease may respond to oral metronidazole and/or ciprofloxacin given for up to 3 months, and to azathioprine or MP in the long term (Table 6.4). Healing of more than 50% of perianal fistulas occurs in about 60% of patients treated with infliximab; however, fistulas often reopen if the treatment is discontinued. Those with suppurating perianal Crohn's disease need surgery, minimized as far as possible (see Chapter 7). In severe perianal disease, however, radical surgery with proctocolectomy may eventually prove necessary.

Crohn's colitis. The treatment of active Crohn's colitis closely resembles that of active ulcerative colitis (see Table 5.1); the differences are outlined in Table 6.5, the main one being the value of infliximab or other anti-TNFα antibody given long term in preventing the need for surgery necessitating permanent ileostomy. Unlike ulcerative colitis, moderately active Crohn's colitis may be improved by oral metronidazole, 400 mg twice daily for up to 3 months, if tolerated, in up to 50% of patients who want to avoid corticosteroids or aminosalicylates. Liquid formula diets may also be effective, but Crohn's colitis responds less well than ileocecal disease to this form of therapy.

In patients who require total colectomy, permanent ileostomy is preferable to an ileoanal pouch because of the high incidence of pouch failure and sepsis in Crohn's disease (see Chapter 7). In rare individuals with refractory segmental colitis, local resection of short diseased segments can be performed.

Toxic megacolon is even more rare in acute severe Crohn's than it is in ulcerative colitis.

Oral and upper gastrointestinal Crohn's disease. Treatment of oral and upper gastrointestinal Crohn's disease follows the usual principles outlined above. Patients with oral Crohn's disease are best managed in close conjunction with specialists in oral medicine. Particular treatment

TABLE 6.5

Specific treatment of active Crohn's colitis

Medical therapy

- Corticosteroids, intravenous (hydrocortisone or methylprednisolone) then oral (prednisolone)
- 5-ASA orally
- Metronidazole orally (for mild cases)
- Azathioprine/MP orally if response can be postponed for up to 4 months
- Infliximab or other anti-TNFα antibody for non-responders

Nutritional therapy

- Liquid formula diet

Surgery

- Total colectomy with permanent ileostomy (ileoanal pouch contraindicated)
- Segmental resection for stricture

5-ASA, 5-aminosalicylate; MP, mercaptopurine.

options include topical and intralesional steroids and topical tacrolimus paste; some food constituents should be avoided (e.g. benzoate and cinnamon). Duodenal Crohn's disease may respond to omeprazole; endoscopic balloon dilation of strictures can also be helpful, but surgery may be technically demanding and complicated by fistulation.

Maintaining remission

The most effective prophylactic measure in patients who smoke is to stop: the risk of relapse in non-smokers at 5 years is reduced by about 30%. The efficacy of drug prophylaxis depends on whether remission has been achieved by medical or surgical treatment.

Strategies for maintaining remission are listed in Table 6.6.

Remission after medical treatment. Meta-analysis shows that, unlike in ulcerative colitis, long-term aminosalicylates have little or no

TABLE 6.6

Maintenance of remission in Crohn's disease

All patients

- Stop smoking

Remission achieved by medical treatment

- Azathioprine/MP or methotrexate
- Infliximab or other anti-TNFα antibody for refractory disease

Remission achieved by surgery

- Aminosalicylates (small-bowel disease only)
- Metronidazole (3 months only)
- Budesonide (for active not fibrostenotic Crohn's disease)
- Azathioprine/MP for aggressive disease

MP, mercaptopurine.

prophylactic effect in this setting. Prednisolone has no routine prophylactic role, not least because of its side effects. Unfortunately, budesonide, 6 mg/day, though less likely to cause steroid-related complications such as osteoporosis, does not reduce the relapse rate at 1 year. In the minority of patients who depend on long-term corticosteroids and in whom symptoms recur whenever the dose is reduced, azathioprine, MP and methotrexate are of proven value in maintaining remission and reducing steroid requirements. As indicated above, long-term infliximab and, if necessary, adalimumab are effective at keeping many patients with otherwise refractory Crohn's disease in steroid-free remission.

Remission after surgical treatment. After resection for ileocecal disease, there is a 50% chance of recurrence needing further surgery at 10 years. In patients with exclusively small-bowel disease, long-term aminosalicylates reduce the risk of symptomatic relapse after resection by about 50%, but the best dose and preparation are uncertain; limited data suggest that at least 3 g/day of mesalazine should be used. In patients with colonic Crohn's disease, aminosalicylates have no preventive role postoperatively. Budesonide, 6 mg/day, reduces the endoscopic recurrence rate by 50% at 1 year for active, but not fibrostenotic, Crohn's disease. Oral metronidazole, 400 mg three times daily for 3 months postoperatively, reduces the symptomatic relapse rate at 1 year, but not beyond this period. Lastly, thiopurines appear to have a prophylactic role after surgery. However, because of their potential side effects and the need for careful blood monitoring (see page 65), many gastroenterologists confine the prophylactic use of these drugs to those with aggressive disease (for example with abscesses or fistulation), after confirmation of recurrent mucosal disease at ileocolonoscopy done 6 months after surgery, and/or after two or more operations.

Follow-up. The rarity with which primary care providers see Crohn's disease, and the wide variety of its manifestations and complications, mean that most patients should be followed up in specialist hospital clinics (see Table 5.1).

Patients with active disease or those receiving therapy need more frequent hospital review for:

- adjustment of their treatment according to the progress of their disease
- monitoring of side effects (see Tables 4.1, 4.3 and 4.4).

For those in remission who are receiving no therapy, follow-up may take place at annual intervals, and may need to include tests to check for:

- occult disease activity (blood count, ESR, C-reactive protein, albumin, fecal calprotectin levels)
- undernutrition (weight and body mass index; serum albumin, calcium, phosphate and sometimes magnesium and zinc levels; red-cell folate; and serum vitamin B_{12} levels in those with terminal ileal disease or resection)
- osteoporosis (bone densitometry)
- other complications of Crohn's disease, such as liver disease (liver-function tests)
- colonoscopic surveillance and biopsy for dysplasia in patients with extensive Crohn's colitis, as for those with extensive ulcerative colitis (see page 98).

Key points – medical management of Crohn's disease

- The treatment of active Crohn's disease depends on its site and the nature of the pathological process causing the symptoms.
- Therapeutic options for active Crohn's disease include corticosteroids, aminosalicylates, antibiotics, a liquid formula diet, immunomodulatory agents, infliximab, adalimumab and surgery.
- All patients with Crohn's disease should be encouraged to stop smoking, given the adverse effect of smoking on the natural history of the disease.
- Patients with Crohn's disease should participate in decisions about their treatment, particularly in relation to the use of new biological therapies or possible surgery.

Key references

Alfadhli AA, McDonald JW, Feagan BG. Methotrexate for induction of remission in refractory Crohn's disease. *Cochrane Database Syst Rev* 2004, issue 4:CD003459. www.thecochranelibrary.com

Cammá C, Giunta M, Rosselli M et al. Mesalazine in the maintenance treatment of Crohn's disease: a meta-analysis adjusted for confounding variables. *Gastroenterology* 1997; 113:1465–73.

Carter MJ, Lobo AJ, Travis SP. IBD Section, British Society of Gastroenterology. Guidelines for the management of inflammatory bowel disease in adults. *Gut* 2004;53 (suppl 5):V1–16.

Griffiths AM, Ohlsson A, Scherman PM et al. Meta-analysis of enteral nutrition as a primary treatment of active Crohn's disease. *Gastroenterology* 1995;108:1056–67.

Hanauer SB, Feagan BG, Lichtenstein GR et al. Maintenance infliximab for Crohn's disease: the ACCENT 1 randomised trial. *Lancet* 2002;359:1541–9.

Hanauer SB, Sandborn W. Management of Crohn's disease in adults. *Am J Gastroenterol* 2001; 96:635–43.

Pearson DC, May GR, Fick GH et al. Azathioprine and 6-mercaptopurine in Crohn's disease: a meta-analysis. *Ann Intern Med* 1995;122:132–42.

Sandborn WJ, Feagan BG, Lichtenstein GR. Medical management of mild to moderate Crohn's disease: evidence-based treatment algorithms for induction and maintenance of remission. *Aliment Pharmacol Ther* 2007; 26:987–1003.

Sands BE, Anderson FH, Bernstein CN et al. Infliximab maintenance therapy for fistulizing Crohn's disease. *N Engl J Med* 2004;350:934–6.

Stange EF, Travis SPL, S Vermeire S et al. European evidence-based consensus on the diagnosis and management of Crohn's disease: definitions and diagnosis. *Gut* 2006;55(suppl 1):1–15.

Summers RW, Switz DM, Sessions JT et al. National co-operative Crohn's disease study: results of drug treatment. *Gastroenterology* 1979;77:847–69.

The management of both ulcerative colitis and Crohn's disease requires close liaison between physician and colorectal surgeon. Specialist nursing care, including that from a stoma therapist, is also necessary both pre- and postoperatively. Dieticians and counselors may also play a key role in preparing patients physically and mentally for surgery and its consequences. Most surgery is undertaken through a conventional laparotomy incision, but in some centers a laparoscopic approach is used for some surgical indications (e.g. right hemicolectomy).

Ulcerative colitis

Indications for surgery (Table 7.1) are as follows.

Emergency colectomy, after appropriate immediate resuscitation (see Chapter 5), is necessary for colonic perforation or massive hemorrhage.

Urgent colectomy is needed for patients with acute severe ulcerative colitis who deteriorate, do not respond to intensive medical treatment in 5–8 days or develop toxic colonic dilation that does not respond within 24 hours to more intense medical treatment (Chapter 5).

Elective colectomy is indicated in refractory, often steroid-dependent chronic active ulcerative colitis, and dysplasia or frank carcinoma (Chapter 5). Occasionally, elective colectomy may be necessary in children with chronically active disease to prevent growth retardation (Chapter 8) and, very rarely, in patients with intractable extraintestinal complications dependent on colonic disease activity, such as pyoderma gangrenosum.

Options for surgery are outlined below and summarized in Table 7.1 and Figure 7.1.

Proctocolectomy with permanent ileostomy has the lowest morbidity and mortality of the available surgical options, is technically the easiest and involves only one operation.

Colectomy with ileorectal anastomosis is useful for older patients with relative rectal sparing who could not cope with a stoma or are

TABLE 7.1

Surgery in ulcerative colitis

Indication

Emergency	Colonic perforation
	Massive colonic hemorrhage
Urgent	Deterioration or non-response to medical treatment of acute severe ulcerative colitis in 5–8 days
	Toxic megacolon
Elective	Chronic active (steroid-dependent or refractory) ulcerative colitis
	Dysplasia in cancer
	Refractory pyoderma gangrenosum (rarely)
	Growth retardation in children (rarely)

Options

Restorative proctocolectomy with ileoanal pouch

Proctocolectomy with ileostomy

Colectomy with ileorectal anastomosis

unsuitable for an ileoanal pouch because of physical frailty or poor anal sphincter function. It is contraindicated in any patient with pronounced rectal inflammation (as they will continue to have bleeding, diarrhea and urgency postoperatively), and in young patients (in view of the long-term risk of cancer developing in the retained rectum, for which annual sigmoidoscopy with biopsies for dysplasia would be necessary indefinitely; see Chapter 5).

Restorative proctocolectomy with ileoanal pouch is the most recently devised procedure for ulcerative colitis, and avoids the need for permanent ileostomy. It is now the favored operation in younger patients (usually younger than 60 years) in whom preoperative confirmation of normal anal sphincter function minimizes the risk of postoperative incontinence of liquid pouch contents. The operation to

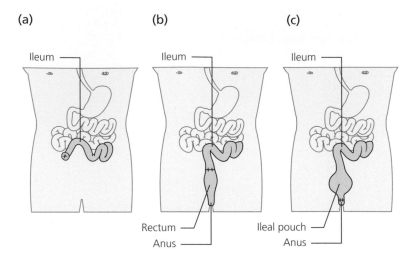

Figure 7.1 Surgical options in ulcerative colitis: (a) panproctocolectomy with ileostomy; (b) subtotal colectomy with ileorectal anastomosis; (c) total colectomy with ileoanal pouch.

fashion an ileoanal reservoir ('pouch') is technically difficult, usually requiring a temporary loop ileostomy that is closed at a second operation a few months later.

Complications of the different surgical options are as follows.

Ileostomy. Although proctocolectomy and ileostomy have the lowest morbidity and mortality of operations for ulcerative colitis, ileostomy incurs a readmission rate of about 50% in 10 years. Complications are listed in Table 7.2: specialist stoma therapists are crucial for their management.

Ileoanal pouch. Complications of ileoanal pouch surgery (Table 7.3) lead to excision of the pouch and conversion to permanent ileostomy ('pouch failure') in about 10%. Early pouch failure is so common with Crohn's colitis that formation of an ileoanal pouch is contraindicated after colectomy for Crohn's disease or colitis of uncertain type or etiology (CUTE). Even in patients judged to have had successful pouch surgery, daytime stool frequency is four to seven, urgency is common and nocturnal incontinence is present in about 20%.

TABLE 7.2

Complications of ileostomy

Complication	Comment
Early	
Skin problems	Rare now with stoma therapists and improved appliances
Adhesive intestinal obstruction	May need surgery
Necrosis, fistulas, retraction, parasternal herniation	Requires refashioning of stoma
Excess stomal output (normal approximately 500 mL/day)	Improves with time postoperatively; avoid salt depletion in hot weather
Late	
Sexual dysfunction	Due to psychogenic factors or surgical pelvic nerve damage
Uric acid renal stones	Due to excess alkaline stomal output

Pouchitis. Villous atrophy and colonic metaplasia occur normally in ileoanal pouches. The diagnosis of pouchitis is made in patients with worsening diarrhea, endoscopic signs of inflammation and histological evidence of acute inflammation with neutrophil infiltration and ulceration. Its etiology is unknown: it may represent recurrent ulcerative colitis in the pouch, or it may be a consequence of ischemia, changes in bacterial flora, or mucosal damage induced by bile salts. About 40% of patients will have at least one episode in the first 10 years after pouch construction. Therapeutic options include metronidazole, 400–800 mg twice daily for 10 days, ciprofloxacin alone or in combination with metronidazole, and topical or oral corticosteroids or aminosalicylates (as for ulcerative colitis; see Tables 4.2 and 4.3). Probiotic treatment with VSL3, a sachet containing a cocktail of probiotic organisms, can be an effective therapy for pouchitis when introduced after a course of antibiotics. However, a minority of patients with refractory pouchitis require pouch resection and a permanent ileostomy.

TABLE 7.3

Complications of ileoanal pouch

Complication	Comment
Early	
Pelvic sepsis	Needs antibiotics, drainage and/or surgery
Anastomotic leaks	Needs pouch tube drainage and sometimes surgery
Adhesive intestinal obstruction	May need surgery
Late	
Poor function	Excessive diarrhea, urgency, incontinence
Sexual dysfunction	Due to psychogenic factors or surgical pelvic nerve damage
Pouchitis	See page 127
Vitamin B_{12} deficiency	Treat with intramuscular hydroxocobalamin
Iron deficiency	Treat with oral iron supplements
Pouch failure	Needs conversion to ileostomy (in 10%)

Crohn's disease

Indications. Surgery is indicated primarily for disease refractory to medical and/or nutritional therapy, or for complications (Table 7.4). In Crohn's disease, unlike ulcerative colitis, surgery is not curative: recurrence at the surgical anastomosis or elsewhere in the gastrointestinal tract is common.

Options. The major principle of surgery for Crohn's disease is to conserve as much bowel as possible; excision of the minimum amount of bowel necessary to remove macroscopic disease is recommended.

In some centers, operations for Crohn's disease are now performed

laparoscopically.

TABLE 7.4

Surgery in Crohn's disease

Indications

Emergency	Free perforation (rare)
	Massive hemorrhage (rare)
Urgent/soon	Small-bowel obstruction
	Small-bowel inflammation refractory to medical treatment
	Crohn's colitis
	Intra-abdominal abscess
	Enterocutaneous, -urinary or -vaginal fistulas
	Perianal abscess
	Toxic megacolon (rare)
	Carcinoma (rare)

Options

Small-bowel disease	Local resection
	Stricturoplasty
Terminal ileal disease	Right hemicolectomy
Colitis	Proctocolectomy with ileostomy
	Colectomy with ileorectal anastomosis (rarely)
	Segmental resection for localized disease (rarely)
Perianal disease	Lay open complex fistulas, drain with seton sutures
	Drain abscesses
	Proctocolectomy (rarely)

Small-bowel or ileal resection. Discrete segments of small bowel are removed with an end-to-end anastomosis. Ileocecal disease is excised with a limited right hemicolectomy, in which the ileum is anastomosed to the ascending colon, with removal of involved ileum, cecum and appendix.

Stricturoplasty. In patients with obstructive symptoms due to very short and/or multiple strictured segments of small-bowel Crohn's disease, the risk of short-bowel syndrome (see Chapter 2) following excision can be averted by stricturoplasty, in which a longitudinal incision of the stricture is sewn up transversely, with consequent widening of the gut lumen (Figure 7.2).

Surgery for colonic Crohn's disease. For patients with extensive Crohn's colitis refractory to medical therapy, the safest operation is proctocolectomy with ileostomy (see Figure 7.1). Ileoanal pouch creation is contraindicated by a high frequency of anastomotic leaks and sepsis, which necessitate its removal. Even in patients with rectal sparing, the recurrence rate is much higher with colectomy and ileorectal anastomosis than with proctocolectomy and ileostomy, making the latter preferable. In rare patients with very localized colonic disease, segmental resection (unlike in ulcerative colitis) is a reasonable option.

Surgery for perianal disease. As in other sites of Crohn's disease, surgery should be minimized, not least because of the risks of inducing incontinence as a result of iatrogenic sphincter damage. Abscesses require drainage and complex chronic fistulas may need insertion of loose (seton) sutures to facilitate continued drainage. Defunctioning ileostomy or colostomy may allow healing of severe perianal disease by diverting the fecal stream, but recurrence after closure of the stoma is common. Strictures can be treated with cautious dilation (to avoid sphincter damage). The threshold for biopsy should be low in view of

(a)   (b)

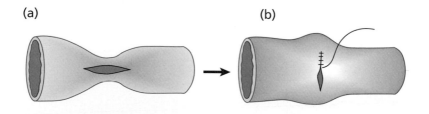

Figure 7.2 Stricturoplasty for Crohn's disease: (a) longitudinal incision through stricture; (b) incision sewn up transversely to widen lumen.

the occasional development of anal carcinoma in relation to chronic perianal Crohn's disease. Proctectomy is sometimes needed for severe and refractory anorectal Crohn's disease.

Complications of removing the terminal ileum for ileocecal or ileal Crohn's disease (right hemicolectomy) are summarized below and in Table 7.5.

Recurrence of Crohn's disease. In about 70% of patients, colonoscopy shows recurrent aphthoid ulceration, usually immediately proximal to the anastomosis, 1 year after right hemicolectomy. Long-term oral aminosalicylates or postoperative treatment with oral metronidazole for 3 months reduces the endoscopic recurrence rate at 1 year, but the effect of such therapy on the symptomatic recurrence rate of 50% at 5 years and the rate of need for repeat surgery of 50% at 10 years is not clear (see Chapter 6). Stopping smoking reduces the recurrence rate.

Bile-salt malabsorption. By removing their site of absorption, terminal ileal resection leads to the passage of primary bile salts (cholate and chenodeoxycholate) into the colon, where they:

- induce mucosal secretion of water and electrolytes (with resultant diarrhea)
- increase mucosal permeability to dietary oxalate (predisposing to enteric hyperoxaluria and urinary oxalate stones)
- cause fecal loss of bile salts (increasing the risk of cholesterol gallstones).

TABLE 7.5

Long-term complications of resection for ileocecal Crohn's disease

Recurrence of Crohn's disease

Bile-salt malabsorption

- Cholegenic diarrhea
- Enteric hyperoxaluria, urinary oxalate stones
- Gallstones

Vitamin B_{12} deficiency

As intestinal adaptation occurs postoperatively, cholegenic diarrhea often improves; in the interim, symptomatic treatment with antidiarrheal agents, such as codeine phosphate or loperamide, or with a bile-salt-binding ion-exchange resin such as colestyramine may help.

Enteric hyperoxaluria is treated with a low-oxalate (i.e. avoiding spinach, rhubarb, beetroot, strawberries, chocolate, tea, coffee and cola), low-fat, high-calcium, high-fluid diet.

Vitamin B$_{12}$ deficiency. After surgery involving terminal ileal resection, particularly if more than 1000 mm has been removed, patients should have annual checks of their serum vitamin B$_{12}$ level, with replacement by hydroxocobalamin, 1000 µg intramuscularly every 3 months, in the event of deficiency.

Key points – surgery

- Surgery offers a cure for ulcerative colitis, but there is always a risk of recurrence of Crohn's disease after resection.
- The patient should be closely involved in the decision to undertake surgery.

Key references

Delaney CP, Fazio VW. Crohn's disease of the small bowel. *Surg Clin N Am* 2001;81:137–58.

Gionchetti P, Rizzello F, Venturi A et al. Oral bacteriotherapy as maintenance treatment in patients with chronic pouchitis: a double-blind, placebo-controlled trial. *Gastroenterology* 2000;119:305–9.

Lee ECG, Papaioannou N. Minimal surgery for chronic obstruction in patients with extensive or universal Crohn's disease. *Ann R Coll Surg Engl* 1982;64:229–33.

Stocchi L, Pemberton JH. Pouch and pouchitis. *Gastroenterol Clin N Am* 2001;30:223–41.

Fertility

Female fertility is not impaired except in active IBD. Because of the risk of inadequate absorption, women with diarrhea due to IBD should not rely exclusively on the oral contraceptive pill to prevent pregnancy.

Fertility is reduced as a result of azoospermia in male patients taking sulfasalazine, but this can be reversed within a few weeks by switching to an alternative aminosalicylate (see Tables 4.2 and 4.3).

Pregnancy and lactation

Outcome of pregnancy is normal in women with quiescent IBD, but there is an increased rate of spontaneous abortion, premature delivery and stillbirth in those with persistently active disease.

Activity of IBD. Pregnancy itself has no consistent effect on the activity of IBD, although the disease occasionally flares early in the puerperium.

Treatment. Corticosteroids and aminosalicylates can be used safely during pregnancy and lactation; withholding them exposes the mother and fetus unnecessarily to the adverse consequences of active disease. Azathioprine and MP appear to be safe in pregnancy. Other immunomodulatory drugs and prolonged courses of metronidazole are contraindicated in pregnancy. Although currently contraindicated in pregnancy, inadvertent use of either infliximab or adalimumab during this period has not been associated with an adverse outcome; both should be withheld in the last trimester, however, so as to avoid placental transfer to the newborn. Surgery is occasionally necessary in very sick women, and is associated with a high rate of fetal loss.

IBD in childhood

Prevalence. Ulcerative colitis may occur at any age. Allergy to cows' milk protein produces a similar syndrome in babies after weaning and

---

Key points – IBD in pregnancy and childhood

- Most women with IBD have uneventful pregnancies, provided they seek prompt treatment for relapses.
- Corticosteroids, aminosalicylates and azathioprine appear to be well tolerated in pregnancy.
- A liquid formula diet is the preferred first-line treatment in children with active Crohn's disease.
- To maximize growth in children, active IBD should be promptly suppressed with nutritional therapy, azathioprine, timely and appropriate surgery and/or infliximab; prolonged courses of corticosteroids should be avoided.

---

needs to be excluded. Crohn's disease is rare in children under the age of 8, but its incidence in this age group appears to be increasing.

Diagnosis. The diagnosis of IBD in children is often delayed. It should be considered early in children not only with classic symptoms, such as pain and diarrhea (see Chapter 2), but also in those with delayed growth and puberty. Prompt referral to a specialist pediatric gastroenterology unit is advised for appropriate investigation along conventional lines (see Chapter 3). Because of the likely lifetime radiation exposure related to investigation of IBD, it is particularly important to use ionizing radiation imaging as little as possible in children (see Chapter 3).

Treatment. The principles of treatment for children are the same as for adults. However, the adverse effects of IBD on growth and pubertal development mean that active disease should be suppressed as soon as possible, undernutrition reversed and prolonged courses of corticosteroids avoided. In pediatric and adolescent Crohn's disease, unlike in the adult disease, enteral nutrition with a liquid formula diet, given if necessary by fine-bore nasogastric tube, plays a major primary therapeutic role. Because of the need to maintain growth and

development, prepubertal colectomy for ulcerative colitis and resection for Crohn's disease are also more frequently used than in adults. Azathioprine is a useful option in steroid-dependent children in whom surgery is inappropriate or declined; infliximab and adalimumab are invaluable additions to therapy in those refractory to or intolerant of thiopurines and/or methotrexate. In all children with IBD, growth should be carefully monitored on weight-for-height charts.

Key references

Barton JR, Ferguson A. Clinical features, morbidity and mortality of Scottish children with inflammatory bowel disease. *Q J Med* 1990;75:423–39.

Connell W, Miller A. Treating inflammatory bowel disease during pregnancy: risks and safety of drug therapy. *Drug Saf* 1999;21:311–23.

Dejaco C, Mittermaier C, Reinisch W et al. Azathioprine treatment and male fertility in inflammatory bowel disease. *Gastroenterology* 2001; 121:1048–53.

Diav-Citrin O, Park YH, Veersuntharam G et al. The safety of mesalamine in human pregnancy: a prospective controlled cohort study. *Gastroenterology* 1998;114:23–8.

Escher JC, Taminiau JAJM, Nieuwenhuis EES et al. Treatment of inflammatory bowel disease in childhood: best available evidence. *Inflamm Bowel Dis* 2003;9:34–58.

Heuschkel R, Salvestrini C, Beattie RM et al. Guidelines for the management of growth failure in childhood inflammatory bowel disease. *Inflamm Bowel Dis* 2008 Feb 11 [Epub ahead of print].

Heuschkel RB, Walker-Smith JA. Enteral nutrition in inflammatory bowel disease of childhood. *J Parenter Enteral Nutr* 1999; 23:S29–32.

Hudson M, Flett G, Sinclair TS et al. Fertility and pregnancy in inflammatory bowel disease. *Int J Gynaecol Obstet* 1997;58:229–37.

Hyams J, Crandall W, Kugathasan S et al. Induction and maintenance infliximab therapy for the treatment of moderate-to-severe Crohn's disease in children. *Gastroenterology* 2007;132:863–73.

Markowitz J, Grancher K, Kohn N et al. A multicenter trial of 6-mercaptopurine and prednisone in children with newly diagnosed Crohn's disease. *Gastroenterology* 2000;119:895–902.

Ulcerative colitis

Mortality. The risk of death in ulcerative colitis is highest in the first year of diagnosis and relates mainly to first attacks of acute severe ulcerative colitis. In this setting, fewer than 2% now die, the principal causes of death being pulmonary embolism, perforation and sepsis. The overall mortality associated with ulcerative colitis is no different from that of the normal population, the risks of ulcerative colitis and associated colorectal cancer possibly being counterbalanced by the non-smoking status of most patients with the disease (see Chapter 1).

Morbidity. Most patients experience a relapsing and remitting course of disease; 70% of untreated patients have flare-ups annually. In patients with distal disease at presentation, extension to involve the proximal colon occurs in about 20% after 10 years. The cumulative colectomy rate in patients with total colitis is about 30% at 15 years.

Cancer risk. The risk of colorectal cancer is increased in those who have had subtotal or total ulcerative colitis for more than 10 years, the cumulative risk being about 20% at 30 years. The prognosis of colonic cancer complicating ulcerative colitis resembles that of patients without colitis. Colonoscopic surveillance programs are widely used (see page 98), but have not been proven to reduce mortality from colonic cancer in ulcerative colitis.

Crohn's disease

Mortality. The cumulative mortality of Crohn's disease is approximately twice that in the general population. Death is predominantly from sepsis, pulmonary embolism, and complications of surgery and immunosuppressive therapy in those with severe chronic disease.

Morbidity. A higher proportion of patients with Crohn's disease than with ulcerative colitis show a chronic active rather than a relapsing remitting course of disease. Surgery is required in about 50% of patients in the first 10 years after diagnosis. Of those having an operation, 50% will need further surgery in the next 10 years, the risks being higher in those with ileal and ileocolonic disease than in those with purely colonic disease.

Key points – prognosis

- Mortality in ulcerative colitis resembles that in the general population, but in Crohn's disease it is increased twofold.
- Causes of death in patients with severe IBD include sepsis, pulmonary embolism, surgery and immunosuppressive therapy.
- The prevalence, chronicity and onset in early life of IBD mean that it represents a substantial burden of sickness both in the community and for healthcare resources.

Key references

Ekbom A, Helmick CG, Zack M et al. Survival and causes of death in patients with inflammatory bowel disease: a population-based study. *Gastroenterology* 1992;103:954–60.

Jess T, Gamborg M, Munkholm P, Sørensen TI. Overall and cause-specific mortality in ulcerative colitis: meta-analysis of population-based inception cohort studies. *Am J Gastroenterol* 2007;102:609–17.

Jess T, Winther KV, Munkholm P et al. Mortality and causes of death in Crohn's disease: follow up of a population-based cohort in Copenhagen County, Denmark. *Gastroenterology* 2002; 122:1808–14.

Loftus EV. Crohn's disease: why the disparity in mortality? *Gut* 2006; 55:447–9.

10 Future trends

Genetics

The continuing research effort to clarify the genetics of IBD is likely to have a major impact on its management in the near future. Identification of the genes involved, and the proteins they encode, will shed further light on the pathogenesis of the disease, and is likely to lead to new treatments. Such information will enable us to identify relatives of index patients who are at risk of developing IBD, to facilitate diagnosis, and to predict the phenotype and particularly the natural history of the disease in affected individuals. Advances in molecular biology are also likely to enable us to identify patients with IBD who are at particular risk of developing colorectal cancer; colonoscopic screening will become obsolete.

Diagnosis

Less invasive investigative techniques are imminent. MRI is playing an increasing role in the diagnosis and monitoring of complications of Crohn's disease, while positron emission tomography may become a useful way of assessing disease site and activity. Serological methods may soon allow the diagnosis of IBD in those with ill-defined symptoms.

Therapy

Improvements in medical treatments will take several directions. First, conventional therapies, such as steroids and aminosalicylates, will become available in formulations that focus delivery more accurately on the site of disease, thereby further reducing systemic side effects. Already two aminosalicylate preparations have been shown to be effective in ulcerative colitis when used in a once-daily regimen, a development which is likely to improve treatment adherence and therefore disease response.

Excitingly, a continuing increase in our knowledge of the etiology and pathogenesis of IBD will inevitably lead to the development of more selectively targeted therapies. Probiotic treatments are beginning to emerge from an appreciation of the importance of the intestinal flora in driving mucosal inflammation; prebiotic approaches may follow. Such treatments will be particularly useful for the maintenance of remission.

Cytokine-based therapies, derived from progressive elucidation of the complexities of the inflammatory process, will undoubtedly follow existing anti-TNFα antibodies into the therapeutic arena for patients with active disease; cytokine-based gene therapy, applied topically to affected gut mucosa, may prove an important step forward in ulcerative colitis and Crohn's disease, as in other chronic inflammatory diseases outside the gut. The choice of treatment in individual patients with IBD will depend, increasingly, not only on the phenotypic expression of their disease but also on their genotype.

Teamwork

Whatever advances are made in the coming years, the management of patients with IBD will continue to require close collaboration between physicians, surgeons, specialist nurses, dieticians and counselors. In addition, a clinical geneticist may need to join this team. Most importantly, the patient with IBD must be looked upon as a person rather than a case; the importance of a holistic approach to the patient and his/her family and carers is becoming increasingly clear. As management becomes more complex and the options more varied, it is essential that the patient remains at the center of the decision-making process. The individual with IBD must be provided with the means to gain sufficient understanding of the illness and its treatment to allow them to be the fully informed final arbiter of therapy.

Useful resources

UK
Ileostomy and Internal Pouch
Support Group
Peverill House
1–5 Mill Road, Ballyclare
Co. Antrim BT39 9DR
Tel: +44 (0)28 9334 4043
Toll-free: 0800 0184 724
info@iasupport.org
www.the-ia.org.uk

National Association for Colitis
and Crohn's Disease
4 Beaumont House
Sutton Road, St Albans
Hertfordshire AL1 5HH
Tel (admin): +44 (0)1727 830038
Tel (info): +44 (0)1727 844296
Toll-free: 0845 130 2233
nacc@nacc.org.uk
www.nacc.org.uk

USA
Crohn's and Colitis Foundation of
America
386 Park Avenue South
17th Floor, New York
NY 10016
Toll-free: 1 800 932 2423
info@ccfa.org
www.ccfa.org

International
Australian Crohn's and Colitis
Association
Level 1, 462 Burwood Road
(PO Box 2160)
Hawthorn, VIC 3122
Tel: +61 3 9815 1266
Toll-free: 1 800 138 029
info@acca.net.au
www.acca.net.au

Crohn's and Colitis Foundation of
Canada
606-60 St Clair Avenue East
Toronto, ON, M4T 1N5
Tel: +1 416 920 5035
Toll-free: 1 800 387 1479
ccfc@ccfc.ca
www.ccfc.ca

European Federation of Crohn's
and Ulcerative Colitis Associations
c/o Micke Lindholm
EFCCA Secretariat
Gropmorsvagen 28
Finland 10520
Tel: +358 40 577 8179
Fax: +358 19 245 0860
micke.lindholm@pp.inet.fi
www.efcca.org
For a full list of European member
associations see www.efcca.org/
e.f.c.c.a_membership/4.htm

South African Crohn's & Colitis Association
PO Box 798 , Fourways, 2055
Tel: +27 11 465 7449
mossies@iburst.co.za
www.ccsg.org.za

Further websites
http://ibd.patientcommunity.com
www.ibdclub.org.uk
www.gastrohep.com

Books
Allan RN, Rhodes JM, Hanauer SB et al., eds. *Inflammatory Bowel Diseases*, 3rd edn. New York: Churchill Livingstone, 1997.

Irving PM, Rampton DS, Shanahan F. *Clinical Dilemmas in Inflammatory Bowel Disease.* Oxford: Blackwell Scientific Publications, 2006.

Jewell D, Mortensen N, Steinhart AH et al. *Challenges in Inflammatory Bowel Disease.* Oxford: Blackwell Scientific Publications, 2006.

Mamula P, Markowitz JE, Baldassano RN, eds. *Pediatric Inflammatory Bowel Disease.* New York: Springer, 2008.

Stein SH, Hanauer SB, Rood RP, Crohn's and Colitis Foundation of America. *Inflammatory Bowel Disease: A Guide for Patients and Their Families*, 2nd edn. Philadelphia: Lippincott Williams and Wilkins, 1998.

Targan SR, Shanahan F, Karp LC, eds. *Inflammatory Bowel Disease. From Bench to Bedside*, 2nd edn. Dordrecht: Kluwer Academic Publishers, 2003.

Index

Note: Only the more significant entries to Crohn's disease and ulcerative colitis have been given references. There will be more minor mentions that have not been given a reference.